ECMO in the Adult Patient

T0262610

CORE CRITICAL CARE

Series Editor

Dr Alain Vuylsteke
Papworth Hospital
Cambridge, UK

Other titles in the series

ECMO in the Adult Patient

Alain Vuylsteke, BSc, MA, MD, FRCA, FFICM
Consultant in Intensive Care and Clinical Director
Papworth Hospital Cambridge, UK

Daniel Brodie, MD
Associate Professor of Medicine
Columbia University College of Physicians and Surgeons
New York-Presbyterian Hospital
New York, NY, USA

Alain Combes, MD, PhD
Professor of Intensive Care Medicine
University of Paris, Pierre et Marie Curie
Senior Intensivist at the Service de Réanimation Médicale Institut de
Cardiologie
Hôpital Pitié-Salpêtrière
Paris, France

Jo-anne Fowles, RGN
Lead ECMO Nurse
Papworth Hospital
Cambridge, UK

Giles Peek, MD, FRCS CTh, FFICM
Professor and Chief of Pediatric Cardiac Surgery
ECMO Director
The Children's Hospital of Montefiore
New York, NY, USA

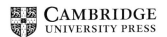

CAMBRIDGE
UNIVERSITY PRESS

CAMBRIDGE
UNIVERSITY PRESS

University Printing House, Cambridge CB2 8BS, United Kingdom

One Liberty Plaza, 20th Floor, New York, NY 10006, USA

477 Williamstown Road, Port Melbourne, VIC 3207, Australia

314–321, 3rd Floor, Plot 3, Splendor Forum, Jasola District Centre,
New Delhi – 110025, India

103 Penang Road, #05–06/07, Visioncrest Commercial, Singapore 238467

Cambridge University Press is part of the University of Cambridge.

It furthers the University's mission by disseminating knowledge in the pursuit of
education, learning and research at the highest international levels of excellence.

www.cambridge.org
Information on this title: www.cambridge.org/9781107681248

First published 2017
14th printing 2022

Printed in the United Kingdom by TJ Books Limited, Padstow Cornwall

A catalogue record for this publication is available from the British Library

ISBN 978-1-107-68124-8 Paperback

CONTENTS

NOTE FROM THE AUTHORS

This book is about ECMO in the adult patient. The adult patient can be defined in many ways but we have arbitrarily chosen someone older than 16 years and, more importantly in relation to the discussed technology, heavier than 20 kg.

We would like to acknowledge the contributions of: Dr Mindaugus Balciunas, UK; Dr Richard Porter, UK; Dr Mathieu Schmidt, France; and Dr Martin Besser, UK.

ABBREVIATIONS

ACT	activated coagulation time
AKI	acute kidney injury
anti-Xa	anti-factor Xa
APR	activated prothrombin time ratio
aPTT	activated prothrombin time
ARDS	acute respiratory distress syndrome
CO_2	carbon dioxide
CPR	cardiopulmonary resuscitation
CT	computed tomography
DCD	donation after cardiac death
$ECCO_2R$	extracorporeal CO_2 removal
ECMO	extracorporeal membrane oxygenation
ECMONet	International ECMO Network
eCPR	extracorporeal cardiopulmonary resuscitation or ECMO-assisted cardiopulmonary resuscitation
ELSO	Extracorporeal Life Support Organization
FiO_2	fraction of inspired oxygen
HbS	sickle cell haemoglobin
HIT	heparin-induced thrombocytopenia
HLA	human leukocyte antigen
ICU	intensive care unit
INR	international normalized ratio

LMWH	low-molecular-weight heparin
O_2	oxygen
$PaCO_2$	partial pressure of CO_2 in the arterial blood
PaO_2	partial pressure of O_2 in arterial blood
PEEP	positive end-expiratory pressure
RRT	renal replacement therapy

A PATIENT TESTIMONY: I SURVIVED ECMO

It is somewhat challenging to define with precision what could facilitate your journey to recovery, as there is no precedent in your life. You are intensely searching for an invisible marker, a destination you seek but cannot see on the horizon.

Meeting with some of the doctors, nurses and physiotherapists who looked after me was a very unique and special experience. Being able to put a face to the names I had heard of so often started to anchor me in this part of my life I could not access before. It also allowed me to say thank you in person, a pivotal part of the healing process, because I was physically there, unsupported by any machine and quite well recovered in fact.

Although without any recollection of the hospital, I suspected that I had probably 'recorded' many sounds of intensive care without realizing it. This was confirmed when I was able to hear an ECMO alarm: the reaction, although slow coming, was strong. This is my only memory, my very own, and I do hold it surprisingly dear. It is an oddly reassuring sensation because it acts as the explanation, if not the actual validation, of everything that has happened since. It almost gives a logical meaning to the last 30 or so months of my life.

Even more noteworthy was the utterly inspired decision to bring me to the bed of a lady undergoing ECMO. This was what I very much needed but was too shy to ask for. I felt overwhelmed and a bit amazed, but I was not frightened in any way. It made me realize how far I had come.

It has proved to be a truly cathartic experience for me. It is vastly important to encourage patients to return, because it is a milestone not only in their journey of healing but in their quest for acceptance too.

Someone told me once that I was brave; I do not think this is true. You either sink or swim. I did not have a choice, that is all. Strangely, it makes things simpler and therefore easier to get on with.

I also believe that you never know what you are really capable of until you are challenged to show it. If you never are, you are blessed, truly.

If, however, the dice is cast the other way, there is still one option left:

Fight back. It is worth it.

Chapter 1

A brief history of ECMO

Starting point

Extracorporeal membrane oxygenation (ECMO) support is a form of extracorporeal life support. ECMO is not a treatment and does not correct the underlying pathological insult. The technology is a direct extension from cardiopulmonary bypass and the heart–lung machine used in cardiac surgery.

Extracorporeal life support technologies include other devices, such as dialysis, continuous haemofiltration and ventricular assist devices

Table 1.1 lists the main events that contributed to the development of ECMO. Early attempts at mixing gas and blood were hindered by thrombus (blood clot) formation. The discovery of heparin at the start of the 20th century circumvented this obstacle. Various devices to allow mixing of gas and blood were developed, with the bubble oxygenator probably the most recognized. In this system, the gas literally bubbled up in the blood. Great attention to the size of the bubbles and the circuit design with traps allowed this to happen without the air bubbles being entrained into the patient's bloodstream and causing an air embolism. The mixing of gas and blood caused multiple disruptions to the blood homeostasis and

Table 1.1 Milestones in the history of ECMO support

Year	Event
1635–1703	Robert Hooke conceptualizes the notion of an oxygenator.
1869	Ludwig and Schmidt attempt to oxygenate blood by shaking together defibrinated blood with air in a balloon.
1882	von Schröder of Strasburg uses a bubble oxygenator to oxygenate an isolated kidney.
1882	Frey and Gruber describe the first 'two-dimensional', direct-contact extracorporeal oxygenator, which exposed a thin film of blood to air in an inclined cylinder, which was rotated by an electric motor.
1916	Discovery of heparin when Jay Maclean demonstrates that a phosphatide extracted from canine heart muscle prevents coagulation of the blood.
1929	First whole-body extracorporeal perfusion of a dog by Brukhonenko and Tchetchuline.
1930s	Gibbon and Kirkland further develop the concept of the oxygenator.
1948	Bjork describes the rotating disc oxygenator.
1952	All-glass bubble oxygenator by Clarke, Gollan and Gupta.
1953	First successful human intracardiac operation under direct vision using a mechanical extracorporeal pump oxygenator.
1955	Kirklin and colleagues at the Mayo Clinic further developed the Gibbon-type stationary screen oxygenator into the Mayo–Gibbon pump oxygenator apparatus, and made it available for commercial use.
1955	Lillehei and colleagues then begin to use the DeWall bubble oxygenator clinically.
1958	Clowes, Hopkins and Neville use 25 m^2 of permeable ethylcellulose (soon replaced by the mechanically stronger polytetrafluoroethylene or Teflon) in multiple sandwiched layers to form the first clinical membrane oxygenator.
1972	Hill reports the first adult survivor on ECMO.
1972	Editorial in the *New England Journal of Medicine* by Zapol: 'Buying time with artificial lungs'.

Table 1.1 (cont.)

Year	Event
1976	Bartlett reports the successful use of ECMO on an abandoned newborn nicknamed Esperanza by the nursing staff.
1978	Kolobow and Gattinoni describe using extracorporeal circulation to remove carbon dioxide, allowing a potential decrease in ventilation harm.
1979	Publication of a randomized controlled trial in adult patients with acute respiratory distress syndrome (ARDS) by the National Heart, Lung and Blood Institute: disappointing results with 10% survival in either group.
1989	Founding of the Extracorporeal Life Support Organization (ELSO).
2009	H1N1 influenza pandemic and data relating to clinical success with ECMO are widely disseminated, including in the lay press.
2009	'Efficacy and economic assessment of conventional ventilatory support versus extracorporeal membrane oxygenation for severe adult respiratory failure (CESAR): a multicentre randomized controlled trial', published in *The Lancet.*
2011	The National Health Service (England) commission a national respiratory ECMO service.
2014	Publication of 'Position paper for the organization of extracorporeal membrane oxygenation programs for acute respiratory failure in adult patients' in the *American Journal of Respiratory and Critical Care Medicine.*

limited the duration of exchange. Interposing a semi-permeable membrane between the air and the blood was a key development that allowed longer periods of support.

The birth of ECMO can be traced back to 1929 in Russia with the first successful reported extracorporeal perfusion of a dog. In humans, the first successful cardiopulmonary bypass was performed in 1953 by Gibbon.

In 1971, a trauma patient survived after being supported for 3 days with ECMO. He is considered to be the first patient to benefit from the technology. A few years later, Robert Bartlett reported the first infant to benefit from ECMO support. Many clinicians were then enthused by the technology and offered it to their patients.

In the beginning

A first trial of extracorporeal support in patients with respiratory failure was initiated by the National Heart, Lung and Blood Institute in the USA. The results, published in 1979, were very disappointing with most patients (90%) dying and with no difference between the groups. The authors acknowledged that ECMO was able to support patients but suggested that it did not stop the lungs deteriorating progressively with no recovery.

As a result, most clinicians stopped offering ECMO.

A minority continued to improve the technique. Others worked on modifying other aspects of the support of respiratory failure patients. Clinicians understood that lungs were being damaged by mechanical ventilation with positive pressure. Methods to decrease this mechanical insult were developed. The so-called protective ventilation strategies are in fact the least-damaging lung ventilation techniques. One promising method was to combine therapies using ECMO to remove carbon dioxide (CO_2) to reduce the amount of ventilation required with mechanical ventilation. However, there was no evidence in comparative studies that using ECMO led to better outcomes than conventional therapy.

Clinicians using ECMO to support infants were convinced that they were saving lives, and several trials and case series proved this to be correct. Paediatric ECMO developed and was embraced by many. Paediatric centres continued to accumulate expertise and experience. But this book is about the adult patient. . .

Enthusiast clinicians teamed together and founded the Extracorporeal Life Support Organization (ELSO) in 1989, justified mainly by the successes observed in paediatric support. This network understood the importance of sharing practice and collecting data from all participating centres. Data about paediatric and adult ECMO were progressively accumulated to inform practice around the world.

Moving forward

At the beginning of the 21st century, technology had advanced with the development and optimization of devices used in cardiopulmonary bypass. The bubble oxygenator had long been forgotten and the membrane oxygenator was being used by all (allowing separation of blood and gas by a semi-permeable membrane). This, combined with the advent of centrifugal pumps, improved the biocompatibility of the whole process. Although still not harmless, the technique was becoming simpler. Improved design removed many mechanical issues. The introduction of smaller, less-intrusive circuits allowed portability. The changes were such that this era can be referred to as the start of the next generation of ECMO (informally called ECMO v2.0).

Specialist centres had started using ECMO in specific patients, such as after lung transplantation. Others were exploring ECMO to support the heart and lungs. The technique was confined to highly specialized centres and the occasional patient.

In 2009, when confronted with a new subtype of influenza virus (H1N1) that targeted mainly young people, the clinical community used ECMO with success to support many patients to full recovery. While it is questionable that ECMO made a difference in outcome (some are convinced it did, but the data have been the subject of many debates), this experience led to a widespread use of the practice. Noteworthy was the fact that ECMO was offered to a large number of very sick patients during the pandemic, without modern health services imploding, albeit stretching available resources.

Simultaneous to the pandemic, the results of a large prospective trial of the use of ECMO in patients with acute respiratory distress syndrome (ARDS) was published in *The Lancet* (the CESAR trial) and fuelled both the controversy about and the use of the technology. This trial showed that transferring patients with ARDS to a specialist centre that could offer ECMO if required led to a better outcome. It did not show that ECMO itself helped.

As a result of the pandemic, and supported by the published evidence, clinicians started to consider ECMO earlier and many providers started to offer it. Some countries set up

national networks (e.g. the specifications of the National
Health Service (England) national respiratory ECMO service
can be accessed online; see Chapter 2).

Parallel to the development of ECMO to support
respiratory function, ECMO has been used to support
patients with cardiopulmonary failure. In this setting, ECMO
can be seen as a way to provide cardiopulmonary bypass
either rapidly (such as in a cardiac arrest situation) or for
several days (such as when continuing cardiopulmonary
bypass after cardiac surgery). Case series (and numerous
case reports) are supporting the development of
veno-arterial ECMO as a way to supply most organs with
a continuous oxygenated blood supply. This support is being
used in an increasing number of patients, based on
clinicians' belief that it helps on some occasions. However,
scientific evidence is lacking.

Key points

- This is a book about adult patients.
- ECMO circuits are now simpler and safer.
- ECMO saved lives during the H1N1 influenza pandemic.
- ECMO is a support modality and not a treatment.

TO LEARN MORE

Gattinoni L, Pesenti A, Mascheroni D, *et al.* (1986).
Low-frequency positive-pressure ventilation with
extracorporeal CO_2 removal in severe acute respiratory

failure. *Journal of the American Medical Association*, 256, 881–6.

Lim MW. (2006). The history of extracorporeal oxygenators. *Anaesthesia*, 61, 984–95.

Noah MA, Peek GJ, Finney SJ, *et al.* (2011). Referral to an extracorporeal membrane oxygenation center and mortality among patients with severe 2009 influenza A(H1N1). *Journal of the American Medical Association*, 306, 1659–68.

Peek GJ, Mugford M, Tiruvoipati R, *et al.* (2009). Efficacy and economic assessment of conventional ventilatory support versus extracorporeal membrane oxygenation for severe adult respiratory failure (CESAR): a multicentre randomised controlled trial. *Lancet*, 374, 1351–63.

Chapter 2

An ECMO service

Staffing

An ECMO service is entirely dependent on its people. The team is organized to provide a continuous service, 24 h a day. Table 2.1 provides an example of a list of the key members of the team. This will vary from centre to centre, depending on local and national organizational factors.

All members of the team require specialist knowledge in managing the ECMO patient, and a robust teaching programme should be established. The volume of activity of a centre should be sufficient to allow availability of the required resources for training. Staff training should be mandatory. Regular refreshers should be provided and competencies regularly assessed. Table 2.2 lists the topics that the in-house training programme should cover. The ELSO provides regularly updated guidelines and resources for the training and continuous education of the ECMO specialist.

The team of educators must be allocated time and resources to attend state-of-the-art conferences. Educators can then ensure their local programme is up to date. Training should include regular water drills, during which a primed circuit is used without being connected to a patient. This allows

Table 2.1 Example of a list of key members of the ECMO service

Title	Role
Lead clinician (ECMO director)	Overall responsibility for the ECMO service. Must practice intensive care medicine but can be from a variety of backgrounds.
Attending clinicians	Round-the-clock management of the patient. These will usually be a mix of post- and pre-certification doctors.
Attending surgeons	Immediate cardiothoracic and vascular surgical support, which is required round the clock.
ECMO coordinator	To coordinate referrals and retrievals. Ensures multidisciplinary education and training requirements are achieved. Develops and reviews protocols and guidelines.
ECMO specialists	Staff who have undergone specialist training and have expert knowledge of the management of the ECMO patient and the ECMO circuit. Will support the ECMO coordinator in day-to-day coordination of the service.
Attending nurses	Day-to-day patient care and bedside monitoring. They are experienced intensive care unit nurses who have undergone additional training in caring for the patient on ECMO. They will be supported by heath care support workers.
Lead perfusionist	Perfusionist with specialist ECMO knowledge who supports the ECMO coordinator in meeting educational and training requirements.
Clinical perfusionists	Provide technical support in relation to the ECMO circuit.
Physiotherapists	Provide day-to-day rehabilitation input.
Pharmacists	Provide day-to-day pharmacy input. Will seek pertinent and updated information in relation to the pharmacokinetics of drugs used in the ECMO patients.
Dieticians	Provide day-to-day dietetic input.

Table 2.1 (cont.)

Title	Role
ECMO secretary	To support numerous administrative tasks related to the ECMO service.
Clinical data analyst	Collection and analysis of data, which is important to develop a strong service. This allows submission to the international registry.
Other specialities involved in the greater multidisciplinary team	Radiologists, haematologists, microbiologists, virologists, biochemists, blood bank specialists, cardiologists, respiratory physicians, neurologists, nephrologists, obstetricians, gynaecologists, clinical psychologists, psychiatrists, orthopaedic and trauma surgeons, ophthalmologists, ear–nose–throat (ENT) specialists and palliative care clinicians.
Ancillary staff	Kitchen staff, cleaners, porters, drivers, switchboard operators, accountants and technical support.

Table 2.2 Specialized topics to be covered in the training of an ECMO clinician

Types of ECMO

Risk and potential benefits of ECMO

Indication and contraindication for ECMO

Pathophysiology of the patient on ECMO

ECMO equipment (including circuits)

Gas exchange on ECMO

ECMO emergencies

Inserting ECMO: Why? When? How?

Liberation from ECMO: Why? When? How?

Coagulation management while on ECMO

The post-ECMO patient: immediate and long term

Complications of ECMO

Cost of ECMO

Transfer of the patient on ECMO

familiarization with the equipment and identification of potential issues. Staff are trained to recognize and manage specific ECMO emergencies, and then do it again and again.

A list of competencies expected from each role for clinicians involved in the management of the patient on ECMO is useful. These can be developed at the local or national level, and the ELSO provides examples and ready-to-use lists.

Multidisciplinary meetings should be scheduled on a regular basis and newly acquired knowledge and experience shared to ensure the whole team continues to learn and evolve.

Doctors

Doctors looking after ECMO patients will require multiple skills. The ideal ECMOlogist would be a surgeon, intensivist, chest physician and anaesthesiologist combined. This person should have acquired the skills of many different specialities. As this is rather unusual, a good ECMOlogist will be a 'connexist', i.e. someone who can recognize his/her own limitations and call on others' expertise. The closest to this ideal are intensive care doctors as they are usually working in this manner.

The starting point for any doctor wishing to learn ECMO is a thorough understanding of the ECMO circuit itself (see Chapter 3). The second key clinical skill to acquire is how to select the right patients, i.e. patients requiring support while recovering from a reversible insult or eligible for another type of long-term support (see Chapter 5).

The ECMO community has a great tradition of supporting each other. These days, multiple courses are available to teach the basics of ECMO. Clinicians involved in ECMO are always willing to help each other.

Adult intensive care skills are central to the safe delivery of ECMO, and all the basics of intensive care management should be adhered to.

ECMO is a complete system of care, not just a bolt-on accessory.

Junior doctors should be involved in all aspects of the care of ECMO patients. The first skill they will need to acquire is to recognize their limitations and when to call for help.

ECMO specialist

The ECMO specialist has a key role. They are immediately available in the clinical area and are the first line between ECMO and the patient. They require advanced skills to ensure no harm comes to the patient. They are the first line in managing the patient and circuit emergencies and, in addition to excellent technical skills, should have effective communication skills and the ability to work in stressful situations.

The ECMO specialist will be skilled in the care of patients on ECMO, and should have a strong intensive care background.

The ECMO specialist must achieve competency through completing the necessary training and assessment. Practical skill sessions concentrate on circuit surveillance, troubleshooting and emergency procedures. Emergency procedures such as air embolus removal are practised repeatedly to ensure competency.

The ECMO specialist can undertake other roles, such as ensuring appropriate anticoagulation, and titrating ECMO flow and gas to ensure adequate levels of cardiac and/or respiratory support.

ECMO specialists can be nurses who have undergone additional training, or can come from other specialities, such as perfusion or medical backgrounds.

All nurses caring for the ECMO patient must have basic skills specific to both the intensive care unit (ICU) and the ECMO patient. They must be able to act immediately in a case of a catastrophic failure of the ECMO circuit. An ECMO circuit must never be left in the hands of a practitioner who is not qualified to look after it.

ECMO coordinator

The ECMO coordinator usually refers to a highly experienced ECMO specialist with clinical, educational and managerial responsibility for the ECMO programme. This person may be supported by deputy coordinators and shift leaders who are experienced ECMO specialists to ensure round-the-clock availability. They are involved in the development of all ECMO-related protocols.

This coordination is an essential part of ensuring the safety of the patient on ECMO. It ensures communication between team members and smooth management of patient referral, transport, cannulation and ongoing care.

ECMO director

The ECMO director is an ECMO clinician nominated to have overall managerial and clinical responsibility for the ECMO programme. The ECMO director does not need to dictate the care of each patient but leads a team to deliver the best possible care.

Perfusionist

Perfusionists are experts in the management of extracorporeal circuits, and their main expertise is with short-term cardiopulmonary bypass used in the operating theatre. A perfusionist will need additional training to gain the knowledge required to manage the ECMO circuit.

Perfusionists are an integral and important part of many ECMO programmes. It is usual practice in some institutions for a perfusionist to prime the ECMO circuit and initiate ECMO before handing management of the circuit over to the ECMO specialist. Once the patient is returned to the ICU and established on ECMO, the perfusionist's role includes circuit or component replacement and transport of the patient to other areas of the hospital, such as the catheter laboratory or the computed tomography (CT) scanner.

A perfusionist who has developed a special interest in ECMO can act as the lead of all perfusionists in an institution and should ensure that knowledge and good practice are shared.

Perfusionists should be involved in circuit design and modifications, management of ordering and stock levels, equipment maintenance and development of protocols.

Transfer team

ECMO is a specialist support that may not be provided in all institutions. A centre will need a minimum number of cases per year to maintain expertise and justify the set-up expenses. Most patients requiring ECMO will need to be transferred from one centre to an ECMO centre.

Patients referred to the ECMO centre will often be unstable, and transfer on ECMO will be necessary.

The difficulty of commencing ECMO on a patient outside the comfortable surroundings of one's own hospital should not be underestimated.

The transfer team will include at least a doctor and a transfer-trained ECMO nurse. The team must be trained and equipped to work in any of the vehicles and with all the equipment that might be used.

Other members of the team

Other doctors, nurses and allied health professionals will be involved in the care of the ECMO patient. It is helpful to try and identify one or two individuals in each department who are interested in ECMO, so that they can develop specific expertise with these patients.

Table 2.1 lists the many specialties required. Surgeons (general, cardiothoracic and vascular), physiotherapists, cardiologists, microbiologists, dieticians, haematologists, radiologists and occupational therapists are all frequently involved in care of the adult patient on ECMO. Specific knowledge will be required from each of them.

Infrastructure

An ECMO centre must be located in an area of sufficient population density to ensure that patients are regularly admitted and a minimum number are supported each year. This number is often the subject of intense debate, but we estimate that expertise and investment will be maintained if a centre supports around 20 patients per year. The relationship between volume and outcome is recognized in many clinical specialities.

The centre must be easily accessible by road, or by fixed wing or rotary aircraft. A helipad directly linked to the hospital is ideal.

The required facilities (Table 2.3) mean that ECMO services will usually be based in tertiary referral centres that can provide round-the-clock cardiothoracic and vascular support, alongside other services such as advanced imaging and specialist microbiology.

The ECMO service will often be part of the ICU, but some centres have dedicated ECMO units. These are specialist ICUs looking solely after the ECMO patient, similar to burns units.

Table 2.3 Co-located clinical services

To be provided on the same site and to be immediately available round the clock	Competent medical practitioner with advanced airway skills
	Endoscopy
	Radiology: CT, ultrasound, plain X-ray, echocardiography
	Access to theatres, including cardiothoracic and vascular
	Transfusion services
	Essential haematology/biochemistry service and point-of-care service
	Haemofiltration and plasmapheresis
	Interventional cardiology
	Physiotherapy
	Pharmacy
	Medical engineering services
	Informatics support
Interdependent services, available round the clock; the response time to these specialities will range from available within 30 min to a maximum of 4 h	Interventional vascular and non-vascular radiology
	Neurosurgery
	Vascular surgery
	General surgery
	Nephrology
	Trauma and orthopaedic surgery
	Plastic surgery
	Maxillofacial surgery
	Ear–nose–throat (ENT) surgery
	Obstetrics and gynaecology
	Organ donation services
	Acute/early phase rehabilitation services
	Additional laboratory diagnostic services
Interdependent services, available during daytime hours (Monday–Friday)	Occupational therapy
	Dietetics
	Speech and language therapy
	Bereavement services
	Patient liaison service

Table 2.3 (cont.)

Related services, available following the critical care phase of the patient pathway	Local hospital and community rehabilitation services
	Specialized rehabilitation services
	Critical care follow-up
	Clinical psychology and psychiatry
	Primary care
	Burns services
	Voluntary support services

Adapted from https://www.england.nhs.uk/commissioning/spec-services/npc-crg/group-d/d16/.

Adult and paediatric ECMO services have historically been combined due to the common technology. It is our opinion that patients are best served in a unit specializing in the original insult (respiratory or cardiac), rather than based on the technology used. An adult patient will not be treated the same way if supported in a paediatric ECMO unit, specialized in the management of neonates or young children with congenital diseases. Local or national organization may influence this.

The minimum specification for the bed space is the same as that required for an intensive care patient. There must be sufficient power points (and these must be resilient in case of power failure). A patient on ECMO may require numerous devices requiring electrical power, as listed in Table 2.4. The ECMO circuit will require a gas supply in addition to that required for the ventilator.

ECMO provides support for many patients with transmissible diseases that may be fatal, so it is important that isolation facilities are available. ECMO centres may have to

Table 2.4 Examples of electrical devices required for a single ECMO patient

---

ECMO console and back-up

Heater and/or cooler

Ventilator

Physiological monitoring equipment

Syringe drivers for sedation, pain control or administration of vasoactive substances

Pumps for feed and other intravenous drugs

Haemofiltration or plasmapheresis machine

Intra-aortic balloon pump

Electric bed

Electric mattress (to avoid pressure sores)

Computer for clinical information system

Warming devices (body warmer, blood warmer)

Hoist and scales

Ultrasound machines

Television, radio, games console and fan (bladeless) to provide comfort to and occupy the awake patient; this may include a power supply to recharge their phone, tablet or computers

---

accept several patients with identical issues (e.g. H1N1 influenza virus or *Legionella* outbreak, or multiple casualties following a blast or chemical injuries). The possibility of grouping patients as a cohort (i.e. isolation of a group of patients) should be available. The team should be trained in using personal protection equipment, and the facilities should allow full isolation. Some centres use personal protection equipment and strict isolation for all newly admitted patients with an acute respiratory disease requiring ECMO support.

The patients need access to an operating room 24 h a day, 7 days a week, and this must be easily accessible from the ICU. Similarly, patients need round-the-clock access to imaging facilities (CT scanner, cardiac catheter and cardiac electrophysiology laboratories). Access to these facilities must be straightforward, with established procedures to minimize mishaps during transfer. All these facilities should be located in the same building and ideally on the same floor (unfortunately, not many hospitals are designed this way).

ECMO equipment needs to be stored when not in use. This requires secure facilities. A technical service must be readily available. It is essential that all equipment is maintained with a programme in place to enable regular maintenance while ensuring adequate equipment is available for clinical use.

For most centres, the majority of patients will come from other centres. Retrieval processes must be in place, including appropriate transport vehicles and trolleys, adapted to the requirements of the ECMO patient (see Chapter 10).

Organization

Clear lines of accountability and good communication are key to the success of the ECMO service. The large multidisciplinary team involved in the management of these patients requires excellent coordination. Conflicting demands must be arbitrated by a clinician with experience and knowledge in the management of these patients. Examples include the general surgeon requiring that anticoagulation be discontinued after a laparotomy in a patient with an arterial reperfusion line or the cardiologist requiring a set of cardiac outputs via a pulmonary artery catheter. The ECMO team must reconcile these differences, assess the risk/benefit ratio between conflictual demands and sometimes make very difficult decisions.

The ECMO service will be intrinsically linked to other services and must have access to a vast range of highly specialized experts. For patients requiring ECMO due to cardiac failure (see Chapter 9), the availability and involvement of heart failure physicians and surgeons is indispensable. These patients may only be able to progress to a permanent ventricular assist device or heart transplantation. For patients with respiratory failure and requiring ECMO, the availability and involvement of physicians with a variety of interests are required. These interests include lung transplantation, interstitial lung disease, chronic obstructive pulmonary disease and vasculitis.

Systemic review of patients on ECMO by a multidisciplinary team happens in the same way as for other critically ill patients. Dedicated clinical multidisciplinary meetings are essential and must be part of the routine of the unit.

As most patients will be referred from other centres, systems should be in place to allow for the triage and retrieval of these patients. Each unit will have appropriate mechanisms to record patient details and clinical reasoning leading to the decision to admit or not and to commence ECMO or not.

The financial and business administration of the programme is often overlooked in this type of book but is increasingly important. ECMO is an expensive mode of support that may be perceived as wasteful by colleagues in other specialities, especially if patient dies after a prolonged duration of support. Data to support expenditures must be collected.

The impact on other services must be recognized. ECMO is resource intensive, and this is sometimes detrimental to other patients, as the ICU facility may not be available or staff may be occupied by the demands of ECMO patients.

Clinical governance should include continuous data collection and analysis. Benchmarking against others, such as reporting to an international registry (see Chapter 15), is important. A review of all patients referred (admitted or not) should be conducted at regular intervals. A registry of clinical incidents should be kept and the lessons learnt shared.

All protocols and guidelines should be easily accessible and regularly updated.

Regular national and international meetings, as well as peer review by other clinicians running similar services, can help to improve quality.

A research programme should ideally be in place. This can range from supporting multicentre projects to multidisciplinary collaboration or in-house complex innovative projects. Appropriate resources need to be allocated.

ECMO centres admitting patients with respiratory disease should be part of a sentinel network to allow rapid detection of new virulent pathogens (e.g. *Legionella*, Middle East respiratory syndrome coronavirus (MERS-CoV), H1N1 influenza virus or emerging pathogens).

Key points

- ECMO requires a multidisciplinary team, with many roles available around the clock.
- The ECMO service must be part of a larger network of services, only possible in large centres.
- A large referral population is required to ensure that the ECMO service maintains its expertise.

TO LEARN MORE

The ELSO website is a mine of information (https://www.elso.org/).

Documents issued by the National Health Service (England) and used to commission ECMO centres in England describe what is formally required to be an ECMO centre (these criteria must be met by any centre bidding to be one of the five commissioned centres in England) (https://www .england.nhs.uk/commissioning/spec-services/npc-crg /group-d/d16/).

Combes A, Brodie D, Bartlett R, *et al.* (2014). Position paper for the organization of extracorporeal membrane oxygenation programs for acute respiratory failure in adult patients. *American Journal of Respiratory and Critical Care Medicine*, 190, 488–96.

Chapter 3

The ECMO circuit

The basic principle of ECMO is to pass blood through an oxygenator to allow gas exchange. If the blood is driven by a pump, the pressure generated by the pump can be used to replace part or all the cardiac function.

When the blood is taken from a vein and returned via a vein, the system is known as veno-venous ECMO (Figure 3.1).

A pump is required to move the blood through the circuit and across the membrane. The returned blood is mixed with the venous blood and then continues as normal (i.e. from vein to right heart to lungs to left heart to systemic circulation). If the proportion of blood going through the ECMO circuit is increased while the patient's cardiac output remains the same, a greater proportion of ECMO blood will bring a higher concentration of oxygen (O_2) to the right side of the heart. If the cardiac output increases while the ECMO blood flow remains the same, the proportion of oxygenated blood that arrives in the right side of the heart will be decreased. Analysis of blood gases in an arterial sample (obtained from the patient) will give the end result of the ECMO blood mixed with the patient's blood, which has passed through the patient's own lungs.

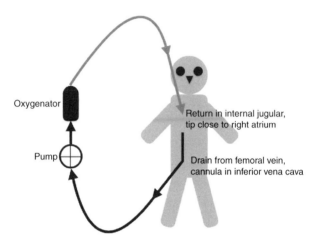

Figure 3.1 Veno-venous ECMO circuit, with drainage from a cannula inserted in the femoral vein (tip in the inferior vena cava) and the return cannula inserted in the internal jugular vein (tip in the superior vena cava, next to the right atrium).

When the blood is taken from a vein and returned via an artery, the system is known as veno-arterial ECMO. The return cannula can be inserted in a peripheral artery (Figures 3.2 and 3.3) or the aorta (Figure 3.4). Alternatively, drainage can be from a cannula inserted in a peripheral vein with the return cannula inserted through the chest into the aorta (Figure 3.5).

In the absence of a pump, the blood would flow in the opposite direction, driven by the patient's own blood pressure. If the pump generates a higher pressure than the patient's own, the blood will go from vein to artery and bypass the function of the heart. This would introduce a shunt with the

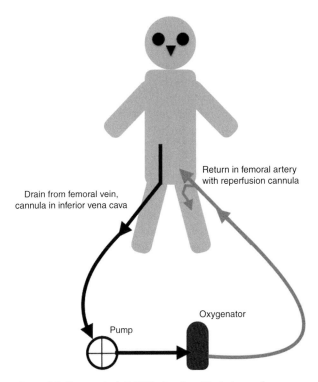

Return in femoral artery
with reperfusion cannula

Drain from femoral vein,
cannula in inferior vena cava

Oxygenator

Pump

Figure 3.2 Veno-arterial ECMO circuit, with drainage from
a cannula inserted in the femoral vein (tip in the inferior vena
cava) and the return cannula inserted in the femoral artery.

injection of venous blood (non-oxygenated) straight into the
arterial system. An oxygenator is indispensable to add O_2 into
the returned blood. This system can then support a failed
heart (by providing the pump support) or a failed lung (by
providing the required gas exchange), or both a failed heart

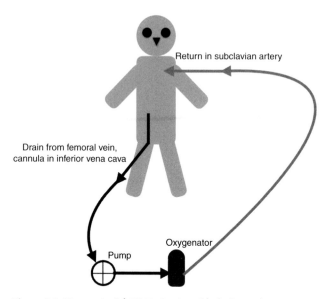

Figure 3.3 Veno-arterial ECMO circuit, with drainage from a cannula inserted in the femoral vein (tip in the inferior vena cava) and the return cannula inserted in the subclavian artery.

and lungs. Of note, the system can pump in line with the normal circulation (such as when a return cannula is inserted in the ascending aorta; Figure 3.4) or pump against the normal circulation (such as when a return cannula is inserted in the femoral artery; Figure 3.2).

Analysis of blood gases in an arterial sample (obtained from the patient) may lead to misinterpretation, as the sampled blood could be coming from the ECMO circuit only, the patient's own circulation only, or both.

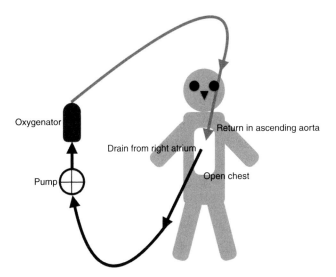

Figure 3.4 Veno-arterial ECMO circuit, with drainage from a cannula inserted in the right atrium and the return cannula inserted into the aorta, through an open chest.

From these two basic approaches, a combination of drainage and access can be configured, including return in both an artery and vein. The chosen configuration will determine what support is provided, hence the mixed (and confusing) terminology of cardiac ECMO, respiratory ECMO, veno-venous ECMO, veno-arterial ECMO, veno-veno-arterial ECMO, etc. We prefer to refer only to the support being provided, rather than the type of ECMO, using cardiac ECMO when supporting the heart and lungs, and respiratory ECMO when supporting gas exchange.

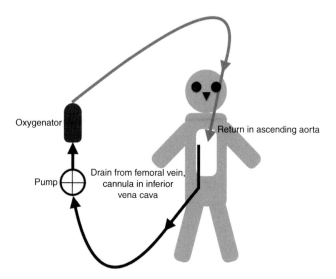

Figure 3.5 Veno-arterial ECMO circuit, with drainage from a cannula inserted in the femoral vein (tip in the inferior vena cava) and the return cannula inserted into the aorta, through an open chest.

Examples of the various configurations are shown in Figures 3.6, 3.7, 3.8 and 3.9.

In the absence of a pump, a veno-arterial approach will become arterio-venous with the patient's own blood pressure driving the blood through the oxygenator. This equates to introducing a new vascular bed through which part of the blood is diverted (blood will be pumped through the liver, kidneys, gut, skin and the ECMO circuit). Gas exchange will happen in the oxygenator.

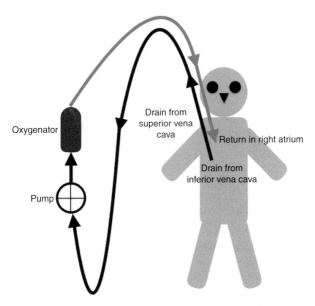

Figure 3.6 Veno-venous ECMO circuit, with drainage from a double-lumen cannula inserted in the jugular vein. Blood is drained from the superior and inferior vena cava and returned via the atrium.

In terms of circuitry, veno-venous and veno-arterial ECMO are identical and this will be discussed further in this chapter. Arterio-venous circuits are discussed in Chapter 13.

The principle components of the ECMO circuit include the cannula (discussed in Chapter 6), tubing, blood pump, oxygenator and heater/cooler (all discussed in this chapter). A diagram illustrating the circuit is shown in Figure 3.10.

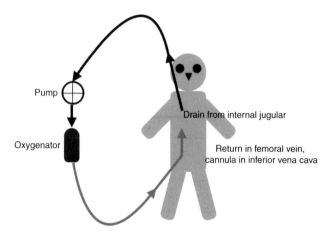

Figure 3.7 Veno-venous ECMO circuit, with drainage from a cannula inserted in the jugular vein and the return cannula inserted in the femoral vein (tip in the superior vena cava, next to the right atrium).

Components of the ECMO circuit (except the cannula)

Tubing

The tubing comprises the pipes connecting the various elements of the ECMO circuit. Blood flows through them and they are joined to other components, such as the cannula and oxygenator. ECMO centres may have slightly differing configurations of tubing, but the basic principle is similar.

The tubing is transparent to allow clinicians to observe the blood colour and detect the accumulation of a thrombus.

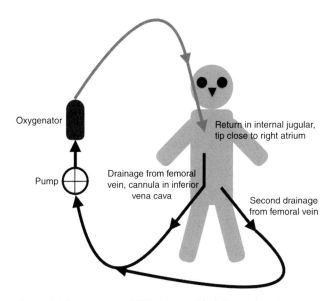

Oxygenator

Pump

Return in internal jugular, tip close to right atrium

Drainage from femoral vein, cannula in inferior vena cava

Second drainage from femoral vein

Figure 3.8 Veno-venous ECMO circuit, with drainage from two cannulas, each inserted in one of the femoral veins (one long cannula with the tip in the inferior vena cava and one short cannula with the tip in the iliac vein) and the return cannula inserted in the internal jugular vein (tip in the superior vena cava, next to the right atrium).

The tubing should be as short as possible but long enough not to impede the patient's movement. Shorter tubing allows for less priming volume and decreases exposure of the blood to foreign surfaces and heat loss. Patient movements include passive mobilization (e.g. transport to the CT scanner) or active exercise (e.g. a patient on a fixed bike). Modifying the length of the circuit is possible but dangerous, as cutting the tubing can lead to air entrainment, blood loss, thrombosis or

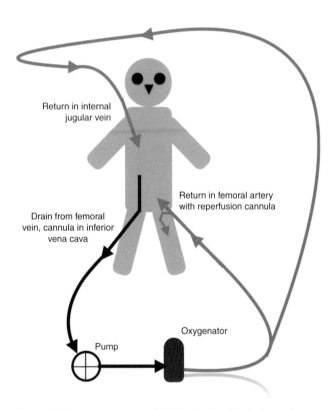

Figure 3.9 Veno-veno-arterial ECMO circuit, with drainage from a cannula inserted in the femoral vein (tip in the inferior vena cava) and the return divided between a cannula inserted in the femoral artery and a cannula inserted in the jugular vein.

infection, as well as subsequent circuit rupture or disconnection.

The majority of tubing is made of polyvinyl chloride. The tubing is often heparin coated to improve biocompatibility,

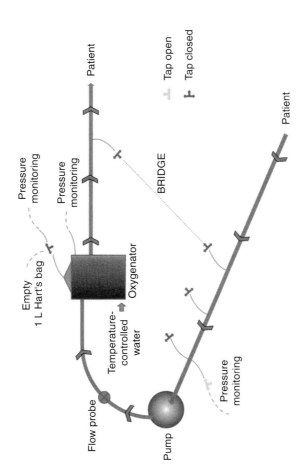

Figure 3.10 Diagram illustrating an ECMO circuit.

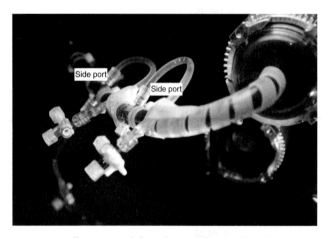

Figure 3.11 Illustration of the side ports that can be added to an ECMO circuit.

reducing the risk of thrombosis and a systemic inflammatory response as the blood is exposed to foreign material. The search for a more biocompatible material is ongoing, and different types of coating are being tested.

By convention, and to allow sufficient blood flow, adult tubing has an internal diameter of 3/8 inch.

The tubes can have side ports (Figure 3.11) to allow access for blood sampling or connection of other circuits, such as continuous renal replacement therapy. The side ports can also be used to give drugs or fluids.

Connections and divisions are areas of increased blood turbulence, increasing haemolysis and thrombus formation.

The high pressures on the arterial (return or after the pump) side of the ECMO circuit limit the use of access ports on this side. Rapid blood loss will occur if inadvertently opened.

The negative pressures generated on the venous side (drainage from the patient with negative pressure generated by the pump) means that air can be entrained into the circuit when accessing a port on this side. Air can cause pump malfunction or even return to the patient. Clear guidelines and careful handling of these ports are required. Protocols should be in place to manage inadvertent air entrainment, and qualified staff should be trained to deal with these situations (practising it repeatedly to be ready for the rare times it happens).

A bridge between the venous and the arterial lines (Figure 3.12) allows recirculation of blood within the ECMO circuit

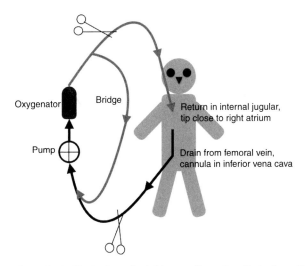

Figure 3.12 Illustration of a bridge configuration that allows fluid to recirculate in the ECMO circuit without entering the patient.

(note: many clinicians wrongly assume initially that the recirculation of blood is on the patient side).

The bridge could, in theory, be used during weaning of a patient from ECMO, maintaining high blood flow through the oxygenator. This is a dangerous manoeuvre, as the blood flow will be lower in some components of the circuit, such as the cannula, leading to the formation of a thrombus. A bridge can be used to recirculate blood while removing air, a technique that can prove life-saving when air has suddenly been entrained into the system. When not in use, the bridge is filled with priming fluid. Bridge tubing not in use should not be left full of stagnant blood.

Blood pump

Blood flow through the ECMO circuit is driven by a pump. Centrifugal pumps are now preferred to roller pumps as they cause less haemolysis and require less anticoagulation. This book assumes you will only use centrifugal pumps.

Centrifugal pumps operate by creating a fluid vortex formed by a rapidly spinning impeller. The impeller is magnetically levitated or spins on a small bearing (Figure 3.13). Magnetically levitated centrifugal pumps require no direct contact between the impeller and the pump housing, eliminating particle or heat generation. This reduces haemolysis and thrombus formation, and has a lower risk of mechanical failure.

The impeller energy can dissipate in heat if no flow is created, but will usually be transformed into kinetic energy.

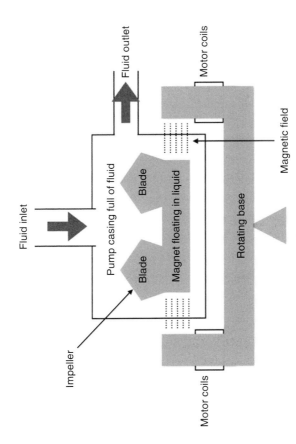

Figure 3.13 Centrifugal pumps operate by creating a fluid vortex formed by a rapidly spinning impeller. The impeller is magnetically levitated or spins on a small bearing.

This creates a negative pressure before the pump, entraining blood from the patient. The blood is then moved forward and positive pressure is generated in the returning limb of the circuit.

Centrifugal pumps are preload dependent and afterload sensitive. This means that the number of revolutions per minute of the impeller will not be the sole determinant of the flow through the circuit. If the circuit is occluded, the pump will continue to spin. If the occlusion is after the pump, the impeller will continue to spin but the pressure will increase.

The pump preload will decrease if the patient is hypovolaemic or if there is any obstruction to blood flow entering the pump (e.g. reduced venous filling due to a tension pneumothorax or kinking of the cannula/tubing). As the interruption is before the pump, the spin will continue but the energy from the impeller will dissipate in heat rather than flow, as no fluid will be sucked in.

The pump afterload will increase if the resistance to flow after the pump increases. This could be between the pump and the patient, such as observed in the case of a thrombus or kinks in the return cannula/tubing, or thrombus build-up in the oxygenator. In veno-arterial ECMO, when the cannula ends are not in the same vascular compartment, an increase in the patient's own blood pressure will increase the afterload, and this in turn will decrease blood flow, even if the impeller is still revolving at the same rate.

Cannula choice (see Chapter 6) will therefore affect the pump flow as the length and diameter of the cannula will create a resistance to flow. In all circuits, the drainage cannula should always be wider than the return cannula to optimize potential flow.

Blood flow through a circuit driven by a centrifugal pump must be continually monitored with an ultrasonic flow meter. The pump speed will be constant, but the blood flow will be dependent on resistance before and after the pump.

Circuits with centrifugal pumps are completely non-occlusive; this means that there is a continuity from one end to the other, without one-way valves. If the pump stops, the blood can stagnate (such as in a veno-venous configuration) or flow in the reverse direction (such as in a veno-arterial configuration as the arterial blood pressure will be higher than the venous pressure, driving the blood from artery to vein). This can have catastrophic consequences in veno-arterial ECMO. The energy generated by the pump in a veno-arterial ECMO circuit must create a higher pressure than the patient's own mean arterial pressure.

Oxygenator

Gas exchange occurs within the oxygenator (Figure 3.14). It is often referred to as an artificial lung, but all astute physicians will know that the lungs do much more than exchange gases. The oxygenator is only a gas-exchange interface.

Early oxygenators used to mix blood and gas bubbles, but membrane oxygenators have proven to be safer and more

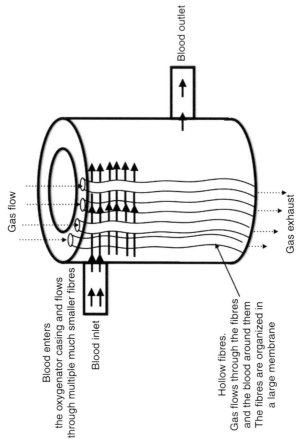

Gas flow

Blood outlet

Blood enters
the oxygenator casing and flows
through multiple much smaller fibres

Blood inlet

Hollow fibres.
Gas flows through the fibres
and the blood around them
The fibres are organized in
a large membrane

Gas exhaust

Figure 3.14 Schematics of a membrane oxygenator.

efficient (the blood and gas are separated by a membrane, allowing only the passage of gas).

Current oxygenators are based on the positioning of multiple hollow fibres creating channels, with the most commonly used material being polymethylpentene fibres. These fibres have better durability and cause less haemolysis. The incidence of plasma leakage is also reduced.

As blood is pumped through the oxygenator casing, the gas (known as sweep gas) flows through the inside of the hollow fibres. The fibre walls (of polymethylpentene) are then the interface through which O_2 and CO_2 transfer occurs.

Oxygenators are made of a case through which the blood is passing and fibres immersed in it, with gas flowing through the fibres. The case will be immersed in a heating/cooling bath to allow thermoregulation.

Gas is delivered to the oxygenator via a blender with a flowmeter that is titrated to regulate gas flow.

In the oxygenator, O_2 transfer is dependent on: (1) the surface area of the membrane; (2) the fraction of delivered O_2 in the sweep gas; and (3) the time the blood is in contact with the membrane. The surface area has been substantially increased by using hollow fibres and should not be a limiting factor in current adult oxygenators. In fact, increasing blood flow increases the number of fibres used and maximizes contact (so higher blood flow usually means a higher O_2 concentration in the blood). This impact of increased surface area is greater than the decrease in transfer related to the blood flowing faster in the oxygenator (faster transit time decreases the available time to transfer). If all the fibres were to be used, decreasing the

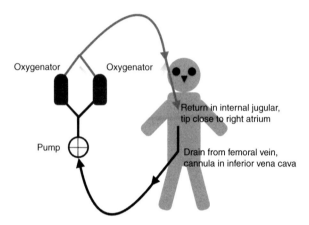

Figure 3.15 A second oxygenator inserted in the ECMO circuit to increase overall membrane surface area. It is important for the blood flow to be maintained at a high enough rate to avoid a thrombus building up in the fibres.

blood flow would probably increase oxygenation, allowing full blood saturation, but this situation is never seen clinically (if one can ever say 'never' in a clinical situation. . .). If all the fibres are used, or too many are out of action due to the presence of microthrombi, a second oxygenator will increase the surface area and improve O_2 delivery (Figure 3.15). The efficacy of adding an oxygenator (in parallel) is disputed, as modern oxygenators are built in such a way as to maximize use of the possible flow attainable with a 3/8 inch tubing. In practice, a second oxygenator is used when everything else has failed. The key benefit is that it gives reassurance that one oxygenator can act as a back-up if the other one was to fail. The risk is the increased number of connectors in the circuit (weak points) and ensuring that high enough blood flow is maintained in all parts of the circuit to prevent thrombosis.

CO_2 is quickly transferred from the blood to the gas, as long as the concentration of CO_2 is lower in the gas than in the blood. This means that CO_2 elimination will primarily be determined by the sweep gas flow. If the gas flow is high, the gas will always have less CO_2 than the blood and a gradient of diffusion will be maintained. The entire dissolved CO_2 can be eliminated in an ECMO circuit and can easily match the physiological CO_2 production.

Condensation of water within the oxygenator will decrease efficiency and the oxygenator needs to be regularly flushed with a high gas flow to remove the accumulated moisture.

Heat exchangers

Heat exchangers are essential to keep the patient warm. Various systems are available, but most are based on circulating warm water around the oxygenator or tubing.

The water used in these circuits can be contaminated by various organisms. While the water is usually not in contact with the blood, these organisms can be released into the atmosphere and may be a danger to the patient(s), staff and relatives. Local decontamination procedures should not be ignored.

A recognized complication is the failure of the heat exchanger (occurring in around 2% of patients). This is not always recognized immediately, as it is often wrongly attributed to the overall condition of the patient.

Heat exchangers allow the control of temperature within a tight, predefined range, such as is required after cardiac arrest.

Heat exchangers also allow cooling of the patient to decrease overall metabolism, leading to less CO_2 production and less O_2 consumption.

Circuit monitoring

The primary goal in monitoring the circuit is to prevent patient complications. The various elements that require monitoring are listed in Table 3.1.

Table 3.1 Monitoring and assessment specific to patients on veno-venous ECMO

Measurement/assessment	Rationale
Blood flow rate (L/min) through ECMO circuit, measured using ultrasonic flowmeter	Main determinant of arterial oxygenation; loss of flow requires urgent intervention
Pump motor speed (revolutions/min)	Adjusted to provide optimum flow; indicator of motor failure
Sweep gas flow rate (L/min) and O_2 concentration	Important factors determining CO_2 removal and oxygenation
Transmembrane gradient (difference between pre- and post-oxygenator circuit pressure) (mmHg)	Increasing transmembrane pressure gradient may indicate failing oxygenator
Post-oxygenator O_2 saturation if patient not achieving target partial pressure of O_2 in arterial blood (PaO_2)	Less than fully saturated blood on 100% O_2 may indicate failing oxygenator

Table 3.1 (cont.)

Measurement/assessment	Rationale
Plasma-free haemoglobin (if available)	To assess degree of intravascular haemolysis
Bedside point-of-care anticoagulation testing (e.g. activated clotting time, thromboelastography)	To allow titration of heparin dosing and guide administration of blood products
Temperature of water bath (warming of blood passing through oxygenator)	To allow adjustment of blood temperature to desired levels
Inspection of circuit, oxygenator and cannula site	Presence of thrombus, fibrinous deposits, air, mechanical problems, infection and decannulation

Monitoring of the circuit is coupled with monitoring of the patient. Monitoring allows troubleshooting of issues, prevention of problems and an understanding of how the patient is progressing. Various pressures and flows can be measured in the circuit but the 'human touch' is important (or visual inspection, to be more precise). Monitoring of other parameters and the patient is discussed in Chapter 4.

Pressure monitoring

Pressure can be measured in three locations in an ECMO circuit as shown in Figure 3.16.

Pre-oxygenator pressure is measured after the pump and before the oxygenator. This pressure will increase as a result of resistance downstream, such as if thrombi have built up in the oxygenator or the return tubing is occluded.

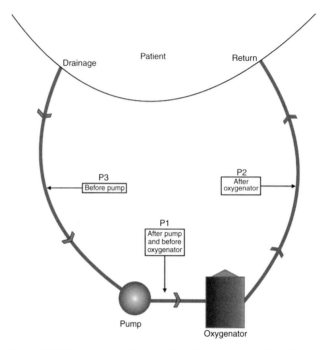

Figure 3.16 Pressure can be monitored in various locations in the ECMO circuit: after the pump and before the oxygenator (P1), after the oxygenator (P2) and before the pump (P3).

Post-oxygenator pressure is measured after the oxygenator and will increase if any obstruction occurs in the tubing and/or cannula returning the blood to the patient.

Pre-centrifugal pump pressure is measured in the tubing before the pump. This pressure will be negative, as the pump is creating a negative pressure that entrains blood from the patient to the pump. A more negative pressure indicates that more force is required to drain the blood. Ideally this pressure will read around –60 mmHg. A value that is more negative than –100 mmHg will increase blood trauma and the release of free haemoglobin. There is a risk of entraining air in the circuit through the measuring port, and some centres have decided not to measure this pressure. It is, however, an invaluable clinical indicator of patient intravascular volume status, and of potential blood trauma. Collapse of the veins on the drainage cannula because of excessive suction should not happen when using this measurement. 'Chattering' or 'fluttering' of the drainage line should not be seen. Some systems (e.g. CardioHelp/HLS; Maquet) have an integral negative-pressure monitoring in an all-in-one circuit (see ECMO circuit selection, this chapter).

The calculated difference between pre- and post-oxygenator pressure is called the transmembrane pressure. An increase in transmembrane pressure indicates an occlusion in the oxygenator, usually due to thrombus formation. The trend should be observed on a regular basis, in conjunction with post-oxygenator blood gas measurements, to detect potential oxygenator failure.

Blood gas monitoring

Blood gases can be obtained intermittently or measured continuously from the circuit and are used to monitor the function of the oxygenator. A deteriorating partial pressure of O_2 in arterial blood (PaO_2) after the oxygenator indicates failure and is sometimes coupled to an increase in

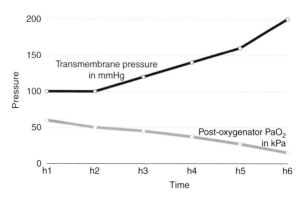

Figure 3.17 Graph showing changes in transmembrane pressure and oxygenation during oxygenator failure.

transmembrane pressure (Figure 3.17). The PaO_2 measured before the oxygenator indicates how desaturated the venous blood is. Measuring the partial pressure of CO_2 in the arterial blood ($PaCO_2$) before and after the oxygenator gives a good indication of the ventilatory property of the oxygenator.

Sampling is done carefully to avoid excessive loss of blood, as the pressure at the sampling point can be very high. To ensure reliable and comparable results, blood gases obtained from the circuit are measured with the sweep gas set at 100% oxygen.

Changing an oxygenator is a relatively straightforward procedure involving cutting the connecting tubing. It is always carried out in aseptic conditions by perfusionists or ECMO specialists. Predicting oxygenator failure is vital to ensure that the change of oxygenator is a planned procedure rather than having to be carried out as an emergency.

In addition to blood gases, other components of the blood that influence circuit management can be analysed. This includes an assessment of the anticoagulation (see Chapter 7) or products of blood degradation. The level of free haemoglobin is a good indicator of stress on the circuit and will decrease with lower blood flow. A higher level of free haemoglobin will often be seen when the suction pressure is more negative.

Flow rate

Total blood flow through the circuit is continuously monitored with an ultrasonic flow meter placed on the return tubing between the pump and the patient.

When the circuit is configured to include more than one return or access cannula, the flow in each arm should be measured and recorded (Figure 3.18).

The flow rate through any tubing should not fall below 1.5 L/min (we advocate at least 2 L/min and usually run the flow at no less than 2.5 L/min). A low blood flow will lead to blood stagnation and thrombus development.

In cases of configuration with multiple cannulas, it may be appropriate to simplify the circuit as soon as the flow can be decreased. (It is better to remove a cannula than to keep flow rates high leading to blood trauma. A venous

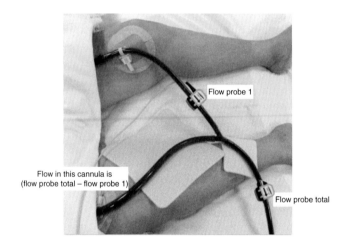

Figure 3.18 **ECMO circuit with two drainage cannulas and one return cannula. Flow probes are positioned so that the flow in each arm can be measured.**

cannula can be removed easily, even when the ECMO is running; see Chapter 6.)

Low-flow alarms may be caused by a low pump preload (not enough blood being sucked in, e.g. caused by massive bleeding leading to the vein collapsing on the drainage cannula, or an intense inflammatory response leading to intense vascular extravasation), a high pump afterload (patient hypertension, a kink in the return lines, a thrombus in the oxygenator) or pump failure, including air being trapped in the pump head. A low flow rate can simply be due to a pump being incorrectly set and revolving at a too low rate. Another reason is the alarm limits being set incorrectly in relation to the required blood flow.

'Human touch' or clinical inspection

Regular and methodical visual checks of the integrity of the circuit and all components should not be underestimated.

The blood colour in the drainage and return cannula should differ when the oxygenator is in use.

The gas tubing should be connected and the gas flowmeter should indicate the correct flow rate.

The temperature of the heat exchanger should remain as set.

Thrombus formation in the circuitry will be noticed first by a nurse conducting hourly routine checks of the tubing and oxygenator with a pen torch.

Kinks or damage to the circuit can be prevented by regular visual checks.

The integrity of all connections and ensuring sutures and tapes are in place can be life-saving. Dislodgement of a cannula can be prevented by regular careful inspection of all sutures (Figure 3.19).

The distinctive sound of air in a centrifugal pump may trigger emergency intervention before any alarms are set off.

ECMO circuit selection

ECMO use has increased due to the developments made in circuit design. Fully integrated systems are now available, rendering training and monitoring easier. Smaller, more compact

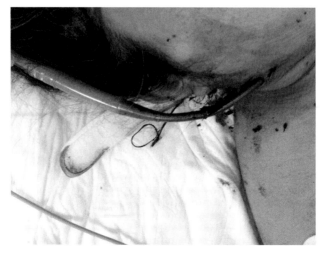

Figure 3.19 Sudden dislodgement of a venous cannula that led to thrombosis.

systems facilitate patient transport and mobilization (Figure 3.20).

All circuits provide the same function, and choice will be guided by cost and training requirements. Fully integrated systems are ideal for units with low usage or high staff turnover. Bespoke systems (Figure 3.21) are suited for units with complex patients or when undertaking complex types of support requiring greater versatility. These bespoke units allow the incorporation of a second oxygenator and the addition of other devices to the ECMO circuit. Some of the pumps on offer can be used as ventricular assist devices. Most of them have excellent safety and longevity records.

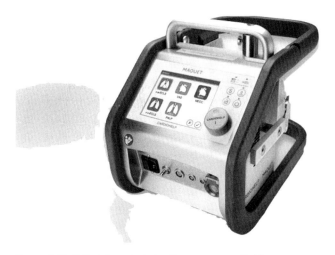

Figure 3.20 Fully integrated circuits are now available.

ECMO circuit maintenance

A rigorous programme of maintenance needs to be in place to
ensure the pumps and other components are in perfect
working order, and sufficient stocks of tubing, connectors and
oxygenators are required.

   An ECMO circuit can be primed with crystalloid fluids in
advance of its use, as long as a strict aseptic technique is used.
This circuit can be kept in a safe area for several weeks.
The benefit of a primed circuit that is immediately available is
obvious in case of sudden mechanical failure.

   Failure is often not an option (back-up equipment must be
available, as mechanical failure may happen even in perfectly
maintained devices). Bespoke systems allow greater flexibility,

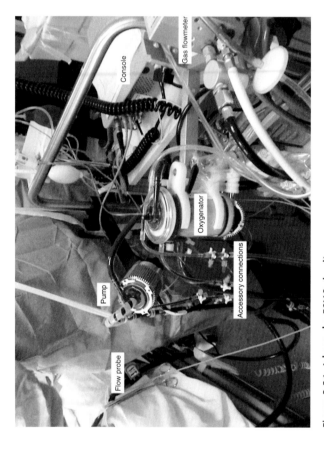

Figure 3.21 A bespoke ECMO circuit.

as only the broken component (usually the pump motor) needs replacing.

Key points

- ECMO circuits should be as simple as possible.
- Modern centrifugal pumps are used in most systems. These are preload dependent and afterload sensitive.
- Monitoring of circuit pressures and blood flow is vital.
- Visual inspection is paramount to ensure circuit integrity.

TO LEARN MORE

Papworth Hospital ECMO Course (http://www.papworthecmo.com).

Lequier L, Horton SB, McMullan DM, Bartlett RH. (2013). Extracorporeal membrane oxygenation circuitry. *Pediatric Critical Care Medicine*, 14, S7–12.

Chapter 4

Monitoring the patient on ECMO

General principles

Patients on ECMO must be managed in an intensive care environment. In addition to the specific elements monitored in the circuit (see Chapter 3), standard ICU continuous monitoring is routinely used.

Bedside observations by a trained nurse are vital. These observations should encompass both patient and circuit. Continuous awareness of the potential issues is important, as a rapid response to events is required to avoid catastrophic consequences.

Standard monitoring will include, but not be restricted to, continuous cardiac rhythm monitoring, pulse oximetry, invasive arterial and venous blood pressures, temperature, respiratory rate and end-tidal CO_2. These will be documented at regular intervals. Hourly observations will include fluid intake and output, and the overall fluid balance will be calculated. Circuit data will also be documented.

Intravascular pressure can be measured in the same way as in non-ECMO patients. Of note, any indwelling venous catheter is a potential source of air that could be entrained into the ECMO circuit due to the high negative pressure.

The position of the cannula (see Chapter 6) in relation to the pressure monitoring may affect the pressure being read. The pressure could be falsely elevated if the cannula and tip of the indwelling catheter are close to each other, or too low if influenced by the negative pressure next to a drainage cannula.

Many invasive monitoring devices (used mainly to assess cardiac output and derive parameters such as extra lung water) have not been validated in ECMO patients and should only be used with extreme caution. These devices have usually not been validated in extreme conditions, and ECMO is not only extreme but introduces a new physiological dimension (which could be called a new physiological bed).

Arterial blood gas analysis will be required at regular intervals and when clinically indicated.

X-rays (chest or abdomen) are useful tools in assessing cannula position and lung recovery (or damage). Ultrasonography, mainly echocardiography, is useful but can only be used intermittently.

Neuromonitoring can be used but interpretation might be difficult. The recorded signals will be affected by O_2 blood saturation and regional blood flow regulation. ECMO and drugs will affect regional blood flow distribution, and it is likely that this will change the way the signal is interpreted. Specific devices, such as near-infrared spectroscopy, only measure what happens in a very small area of the brain, and generalization of the reading is not possible. Moreover, normal ranges are not defined.

Transcranial Dopplers can be used, but it is unclear how they affect management and outcome.

All standard principles will apply, but the clinician has to integrate the extracorporeal gas exchange in the interpretation of all changes. Specifics to veno-venous or veno-arterial ECMO are described below.

Distal arterial perfusion and venous drainage can be affected by ECMO cannulas. Most common is the lack of perfusion of the limb distal to the insertion of an arterial cannula, and hence the use of reperfusion lines (see Chapter 6). Oedema can occur if venous drainage is impaired. Careful observation is required, as the consequences can be devastating (loss of a limb, or even cerebral oedema when the flow through the internal jugular is impaired).

Monitoring the patient on veno-venous ECMO

In veno-venous ECMO, the blood is taken from and returned into the venous circulation. The end result is a venous blood with higher O_2 and lower CO_2 content entering the pulmonary circulation. The blood will mix with the patient's blood that is not going through the ECMO circuit. The final content of the venous blood entering the heart will be based on the admixture of both ECMO and native circulation.

This means that a higher cardiac output will increase the proportion of patient's native (non-EMCO) blood in the final mix; while higher ECMO flow will increase the proportion of 'ECMOed' blood in the final mix. This explains in part why higher ECMO flow brings higher oxygenation!

A final mix with higher O_2 content will affect hypoxic vasoconstriction (but the extent of this, in the context of critically ill patients receiving multiple drugs is unknown).

Oxygen content will be a result of both the blood returned by the ECMO circuit and the patient's own vascular beds.

Changes in ventilation and perfusion will affect the end-tidal CO_2.

When on veno-venous ECMO, most of the monitoring will be directed to observing the recovery of the lungs to ensure that they are not further damaged.

The suction of venous blood is likely to affect any system derived on thermodilution and caution should be exerted when using techniques relying on a venous injectate. Observing the distribution of the contrast dye injected during a CT scan with contrast clearly illustrates that an unknown and variable quantity of diluent is sucked into the ECMO circuit (and returned with some delay).

In veno-venous ECMO, one of the key issues is recirculation of oxygenated blood around the ECMO circuit itself. This happens when the drainage and return cannula are too close to each other, or are located in such a way that the oxygenated blood will be preferentially returned to the ECMO circuit rather than the right heart circulation. The efficiency of the ECMO will decrease substantially as the blood will be saturated in O_2 and low in CO_2, and the ECMO will in effect support the ECMO. Changes in the

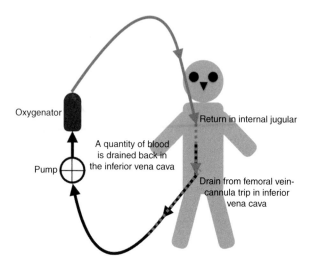

Oxygenator

Return in internal jugular

A quantity of blood
is drained back in
the inferior vena cava

Pump

Drain from femoral vein-
cannula trip in inferior
vena cava

Figure 4.1 Illustration of recirculation in a patient on veno-venous ECMO. The oxygenated blood returned to the patient is immediately aspirated by the ECMO circuit.

patient physiology during support may increase or decrease the amount of blood being recirculated. Dramatic changes can be seen when observing the colour of the blood in the circuit but more subtle ones require the PaO2 to be measured in the circuit before the oxygenator. This value will however vary according to the patient's own O_2 extraction and other physiological changes, and is therefore sometimes difficult to detect. Confirmation of recirculation will often require careful mobilization of the cannula. Recirculation is illustrated in Figures 4.1 and 4.2.

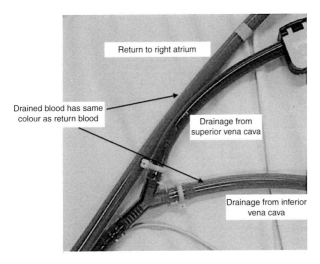

Return to right atrium

Drained blood has same colour as return blood

Drainage from superior vena cava

Drainage from inferior vena cava

Figure 4.2 In a system with two drainage cannulas, it is obvious that the blood in one drainage tubing has the same colour as the blood returned to the patient, indicating recirculation.

Monitoring the patient on veno-arterial ECMO

In veno-arterial ECMO, the blood is taken from the venous circulation and returned to the arterial circulation. The end result is arterial blood with a higher O_2 and lower CO_2 content entering the systemic circulation.

Veno-arterial ECMO bypasses the cardiopulmonary circulation, and the risk of no flow in the pulmonary vessels is high. This may lead to thrombosis. In the absence of left ventricular ejection (which often occurs if the heart is weakened and its afterload is increased by the pressure

Table 4.1 Possible reasons for changes in arterial pressure waveform in a patient on veno-arterial ECMO

Decreased pulsatility	Increased pump flow
	Decreased heart contractility
	Pericardial collection
	Hypovolaemia
	Pneumothorax
	Aortic valve thrombosis
Increased pulsatility	Decreased pump flow
	Increased heart contractility

generated by the ECMO), ventricular cavities will distend and thrombi are likely to be formed. It is therefore important to ensure that there is continuous blood flow through the lungs and no stagnation of blood in the cardiac cavities. Ensuring opening of the aortic valve is required, and this can usually be observed on the pressure waveform. Using a pulmonary artery catheter allows continuous monitoring of pulmonary blood flow. Changes in the pressure waveforms must be recorded and discussed, as they will reflect a change in one of many aspects in the patient's care. The reasons for changes in the arterial pressure waves are listed in Table 4.1.

If the patient is still pumping blood through the native circulation, the blood exiting the cardiopulmonary circulation ('native' blood) will mix with that pumped through the ECMO circuit. The 'native' blood will be more or less oxygenated, and CO_2 will have been more or less cleared, depending on the conditions of the lungs. Both the ECMO and the 'native' blood will meet and mix, but this will be affected by many physiological variables.

If the patient's cardiac output is increasing but the lungs are not functioning properly, the proportion of poorly oxygenated blood will increase (assuming the ECMO flow remains the same, although this will usually not be the case, as a better cardiac function will increase systemic pressure and this in turn will decrease ECMO flow if the pump energy is not increased). The flow distribution is such that some areas may receive hypoxic blood, while others may be hyperoxic.

A patient can appear to be very well oxygenated (i.e. be pink and have a high measured PaO_2) but have an ischaemic electrocardiogram (ECG). This will happen when the blood exiting the cardiopulmonary circulation and entering the coronary arteries has not been properly oxygenated, while the very well oxygenated ECMO blood is distributed in all other vascular beds except the coronaries. A patient can appear bicoloured (called harlequin syndrome) when part of the circulation is supplied by poorly oxygenated 'native' blood and the rest by ECMO blood. This will happen, for example, in patients with peripheral veno-arterial ECMO where the blood is returned in the femoral artery. The blood from the ECMO circulates in the lower portion of the body, while the blood pumped by the heart circulates in the upper portion. On some occasions, a demarcation line can be observed. Arterial blood gases taken at various locations will give values of PaO_2 that can be very different. Of note, interrupting the sweep gas in a veno-arterial circuit (something that should NEVER be done) will inject blood with a low O_2 content and a reverse harlequin effect could be seen.

In veno-arterial ECMO, venous O_2 content will be related to O_2 extraction (itself affected by O_2 content in the arterial circulation). Venous saturation can be monitored, but the clinician has to understand that this value will be affected by many variables (mixed venous oxygen saturation (SvO_2) is always affected by many variables, even in non-EMCO patients) and must be interpreted with caution.

Bypassing the cardiopulmonary circulation will affect pulmonary blood flow. This will affect pulmonary artery pressures. Similarly, the end-tidal CO_2 will be affected by the quantity of blood entering the lung and where it flows (areas that are ventilated or not). The pulmonary capillary wedge pressure can be measured, although great caution is advised in the anticoagulated patient. The variation in pulmonary and intracardiac blood flow is likely to impact on the validity of the measured pressures, but trends can be useful.

In veno-arterial ECMO, there is no recirculation of oxygenated blood in the ECMO circuit itself.

Echocardiography is useful, although it only provides intermittent monitoring of cardiac recovery. Repeated transoeosophageal examination can lead to trauma, and transthoracic examination is preferred. While many indices can be measured, the most useful are still a subjective assessment of function and visualization of valve opening.

Measuring non-invasive pressures may not be possible in the patient with veno-arterial ECMO and with absence of pulsatility. In these cases, sphygmomanometry and a Doppler to detect blood flow are used.

Key points

- Patient monitoring is at least the same as in all patients in the ICU.
- Veno-arterial ECMO impact on standard monitored values is highly complex.
- There is no reliable way to measure cardiac output while on ECMO.
- Neuromonitoring is not standardized for the ECMO patient.

TO LEARN MORE

Chung M, Shiloh AL, Carlese A. (2014). Monitoring of the adult patient on venoarterial extracorporeal membrane oxygenation. *Scientific World Journal*, 2014, 393258.

Chapter 5

Case selection

Introduction

ECMO is a support modality that buys time. During that time, the patient can be treated. If the patient recovers, ECMO has provided a bridge to recovery. If treatment fails, or if no treatment is available and recovery is not expected, ECMO provides a bridge to further treatment or support. Patients with cardiac failure can be bridged to another device or to a heart transplant. Patients with respiratory failure can only be bridged to a lung transplant, as long-term support devices are not yet available.

Selection of patients who will ultimately benefit from ECMO is crucial to the success of a service. Failure to select patients who will either recover or be suitable for further therapies will cause a lot of suffering. Patients will remain for weeks in intensive care with no prospect of recovery. Staff will lose morale by having to care for futile patients. Managers will question the high cost when assessed against outcome.

Sadly, many patients are referred too late for consideration by the ECMO team. ECMO is not a miracle machine and cannot reverse the irreversible.

In the absence of clearly recognized criteria backed up by evidence, the clinician will often have to rely on expertise and experience. ECMO can kill even when patient selection is perfect, or can cause major harm with life-changing injuries. The good clinician will remain fearful, wondering if the timing of starting is absolutely right, as there are no definite indicators.

For all these reasons, most programmes require more than one person to be involved in making the decision to support or not.

Respiratory diseases

The clinician will face multiple factors when considering a patient with acute severe respiratory failure. Potential recovery will be obvious in many conditions, such as acute infection (e.g. *Legionella pneumoniae*, H1N1 influenza pneumonia, aspiration) or status asthmaticus.

An underlying respiratory condition may undermine the prospect of recovery, but this is not always easy to predict. A patient with mild emphysema may suffer a bad bout of flu and recover unscathed after a few days, while others might end up condemned to the ventilator for ever.

Co-morbidities, previously existing or newly acquired, will weigh in when deciding whether to go ahead or not. Constant progress and a team daring to challenge current clinical wisdom keep pushing the boundaries of what will be successful.

Too often, the underlying diagnosis is unknown when life or death decisions must be taken, and inevitably some conditions that appear to be reversible will prove ineluctable. Plans must be made for the patient, relatives and team to cope with this.

The chosen treatment and support modalities instituted because of or during ECMO may transform a potentially reversible condition into an irreversible one. Examples include mismanagement of mechanical ventilation or incorrect choice of antibiotics.

Reversibility

There is not yet a score that allows prediction with certitude of the recovery of any patient presenting with acute severe respiratory failure.

Patients presenting with acute infective pneumonia will usually recover if appropriate antibiotics and/or antiviral drugs are given early. Similarly, patients with acute severe asthma of allergic origin will recover if the trigger is removed. Patients with acute vasculitis or infiltrative disease of immune origin can recover if the diagnosis is made promptly and treatment given accordingly.

Immunosuppressed patients may not have the ability to fight the cause of the failure, and ECMO will not change the course of the disease. It is incredibly difficult to assess the immune system, and clinicians will be torn between the desire to try to save a life by gaining more time and the risk of potential harm.

Transplant centres are repeatedly reporting reversibility of acute rejection, justifying ECMO in immunosuppressed transplant patients presenting with this condition. This often requires great clinical acumen, as immunosuppression and other treatments have to be continuously adapted in this group of patients, balancing carefully the risk or spread of infection and the containment of rejection.

Patients with human immunodeficiency virus infection presenting with an acute severe respiratory failure should be considered. The CD4 cell count helps to predict outcome, but this is not absolute. However, patients with acquired immunodeficiency disease (AIDS; stage 4 of the disease) will most likely not have the immune reserve to control the pathological process.

Many lung diseases are not reversible, including lung fibrosis, emphysema, cystic fibrosis and chronic obstructive pulmonary disease. However, an acute infection may just be recoverable with the possibility that the patient's condition will return to baseline or slightly worsen after ECMO support. The clinician will have to assess the impact of 'slightly worse' and weigh up the probability of a good outcome versus failure to recover.

Specific considerations

ECMO clinicians are eager to have clearly defined selection criteria. Selection criteria have been used in trials (such as the CESAR trial; see Table 5.1) and are used by many centres, such as the national respiratory ECMO service in England. These criteria are interpreted loosely as clinicians are confronted with previously healthy patients and encouraged by previous results.

Age is no longer recognized as an accurate indicator of outcome, and an index of frailty should be used. A reliable

Table 5.1 Eligibility of patients with severe acute respiratory failure, as used in the CESAR trial

Inclusion
Reversibility
18–65 years of age
Murray score (see Table 5.2) ≥3
Non-compensated hypercapnia with pH <7.2
Exclusion
Ventilated with fraction of inspired oxygen (FiO_2) >80% or peak airway pressure >30 cmH$_2$O for more than 7 days
Severe trauma within last 24 h, intracranial bleeding and any other contraindication to limited heparinization
Moribund and any contraindication to continuing active treatment

index of frailty has yet to be published (and is likely to include age but alongside other parameters).

The duration of ventilation is directly linked to the duration of support and outcome, but these vary from disease to disease and depend on co-morbid status. Waking and mobilizing patients on ECMO changes the duration of support and the ability to recover. A patient can be woken up while on ECMO and extubated, or can breathe through a tracheostomy. This allows mobilization and intensive rehabilitation, improving outcome and long-term recovery.

The Murray score gives an indication of disease severity but not necessarily of the chance of survival (Table 5.2).

Patients with cerebral haemorrhage would not have been offered ECMO support a few years ago, and those developing cerebral haemorrhage while on support would have been palliated. This is now challenged, as new veno-venous circuits

Table 5.2 Murray score for acute lung injury

Characteristic	Score
Chest X-ray	
No alveolar consolidation	0
Alveolar consolidation confined to one quadrant	1
Alveolar consolidation confined to two quadrants	2
Alveolar consolidation confined to three quadrants	3
Alveolar consolidation confined to four quadrants	4
Hypoxaemia	
$PaO_2/FiO_2 \geq 300$ mmHg	0
PaO_2/FiO_2 225–299 mmHg	1
PaO_2/FiO_2 175–224 mmHg	2
PaO_2/FiO_2 100–174 mmHg	3
$PaO_2/FiO_2 <100$ mmHg	4
PEEP	
PEEP ≤ 5 cmH$_2$O	0
PEEP 6–8 cmH$_2$O	1
PEEP 9–11 cmH$_2$O	2
PEEP 12–14 cmH$_2$O	3
PEEP ≥ 15 cmH$_2$O	4
Respiratory system compliance	
Compliance ≥ 80 mL/cmH$_2$O	0
Compliance 60–79 mL/cmH$_2$O	1
Compliance 40–59 mL/cmH$_2$O	2
Compliance 20–39 mL/cmH$_2$O	3
Compliance <19 mL/cmH$_2$O	4

The total score is attained by dividing the values obtained from the initial analysis by the number of elements used for the analysis. A score of zero indicates no lung injury. PaO_2, partial pressure of O_2 in arterial blood; FiO_2, fraction of inspired oxygen; PEEP, positive end-expiratory pressure.

can be used for long periods (weeks) without anticoagulation and with minimum trauma to the blood. Many patients with an intracranial bleed have now been supported to full recovery. This extends to other causes of haemorrhage, and ECMO can be used in the trauma patient if the source of bleeding has been controlled.

Frailty

It may be paradoxical to claim that a patient has to be fit enough to survive the major insult leading to acute severe respiratory failure. The patient may indeed not be fit when presenting for ECMO. The physiological reserve will impact on how the patient will sustain the multiple insults linked to both support and treatment.

It is well recognized that modern medicine is increasingly treating older patients who benefit from multiple interventions or adjustments to maintain their health. Drugs given to control blood pressure and heart function may affect renal function but with no direct obvious impact until this finely tuned physiology is disturbed. Severe illness neuropathy or myopathy may lead to so much muscular loss that mobility becomes impaired leading to further problems. Scarring of lung tissue may result in an insufficient functioning lung volume and the inability to recover when the initial disease has been controlled.

Age in itself is not a definite indicator, but it is known that physiological reserve decreases with age. Registries have shown that a prolonged duration of ECMO support is needed in older patients, and poorer outcomes are reported for patients older than 65 years.

Patients requiring heavy nursing care in their day-to-day life will be poor candidates as they are unlikely to recover any autonomy. At best, they would return to their previous status, but sadly this is the exception.

The difficulty in assessing frailty, coupled with the progress made in supporting sicker patients, supports the importance of detailed history taking and physical assessment before starting support. The clinician will be eager that all patients who may benefit from ECMO will receive it, but will want to avoid causing unnecessary harm and inappropriate use of resources by commencing ECMO in some patients.

Obesity

Obesity was previously thought to negatively predict survival, but this has been disproven. While challenging for the ECMO team, morbidly obese patients can be supported with success. Limitations in care are usually due to other factors, such as unavailability of adequate transport equipment, the impossibility of entering a CT scanner and complications caused by physical difficulties mobilizing patients when in bed.

Brain injury

Brain injury is not a contraindication to ECMO, as long as recovery is expected.

Currently, veno-venous ECMO circuits can run for long periods of time without anticoagulation, and many patients with a cerebral haemorrhage have been supported to full recovery.

Duration of ventilation

Mechanical ventilation using positive pressure is detrimental to lung recovery. Studies have repeatedly shown that high-volume, high-pressure ventilation leads to poorer outcomes. The duration effect is well characterized, but one would logically infer that the longer it goes on, the worse it will be. Data also show that starting ECMO at a later stage leads to poorer outcomes.

Many guidelines suggest that patients should have been ventilated for fewer than 10 days to have a chance of recovery. However, they often mitigate such statements by adding that it is acceptable to take on patients ventilated for longer periods but at reasonable volumes and/or pressures.

One approach is to agree that fewer than 7 days of ventilation is acceptable. Any longer periods of time require estimation of the amount of lung that can be saved. This estimation is fraught with difficulties, and there are no defined rules to follow.

Failure of conventional management

It is a widespread misconception that a patient cannot be referred for ECMO before all other methods of conventional ventilation have been attempted. While ECMO carries an iatrogenic risk, it can only be beneficial if the patient can still be bridged to recovery or transplant. Delaying referral or commencement of ECMO to attempt another modality is not wise.

The CESAR trial, a randomized controlled ECMO trial in adult respiratory patients, showed that moving the patient to a centre providing ECMO was beneficial (although the study did not show that the survival of patients supported by ECMO was better). Transport of the patient is a difficult and dangerous time, and is better attempted before last ditch treatment has failed.

Irreversibility and lung transplantation

The question of reversibility is a moot point as patients whose lungs do not recover could be bridged to lung transplant. Issues arise immediately when this is evoked, as multiple conditions must be met:

- The patient has to be eligible for lung transplant.
- The patient will compete against other patients on the waiting list, and will need to be prioritized as they are using precious and expensive resources while on ECMO.
- Organ availability means that long waiting times are often expected. This is compounded by the build-up of antibodies if transfused when on ECMO.

Data have shown that the outcomes of patients transplanted from ECMO are worse than those of patients who have been waiting at home. Many now argue that patient care while on

ECMO has improved since these results were published, and patients awaiting transplant can now be woken up and receive intensive rehabilitation while on ECMO, improving fitness and increasing physiological reserve, in turn improving the chance of surviving the transplant operation.

Some centres have developed strategies by which they offer ECMO support to patients already on the waiting list and progressing to end-stage respiratory failure. Elective commencement of ECMO allows them to wait while awake, exercising and spending time with their family, albeit in the confines of an acute care environment. This concept is intriguing, as one has to be on the waiting list to be accepted, while others who are too fit to even be considered for lung transplantation will not be accepted for ECMO after an acute disease. Ethical dilemma and debate are a constant feature when offering ECMO to patients.

Cardiac diseases

As with respiratory disease, the clinician will face multiple factors when considering a patient with acute severe cardiac failure.

Potential recovery is usually not obvious except in the rare cases of intoxication (such as with β-blockers or calcium antagonists). Patients suffering major intoxication with the drugs listed in Table 5.3 have been successfully bridged to recovery, and it is likely that this can be achieved with other drugs.

Common scenarios of patients requiring ECMO support include: (1) patients with cardiac arrest requiring prolonged

Table 5.3 Drugs where patients presenting with acute intoxication have been successfully bridged to recovery with ECMO

Flecainide
Tricyclic antidepressants
β-Adrenergic-receptor antagonists
Calcium-channel antagonists
Digoxin
Bupropion

---

cardiopulmonary resuscitation (CPR) and for whom the cause might be reversible; (2) patients with intractable arrhythmias requiring haemodynamic support while the arrhythmia is treated; (3) patients with an acute mechanical defect that may be amenable to surgery; (4) patients eligible for transplantation or mechanical assist devices when these are not immediately available; (5) patients unable to be weaned from cardiopulmonary bypass or with major cardiogenic shock in the immediate post-operative period; (6) patients with primary graft dysfunction after heart transplantation; and (7) patients with non-determined problems who can be supported by cardiorespiratory support while awaiting a solution.

Similarly to respiratory diseases, co-morbidities, whether previously existing or newly acquired, will impact on the decision to go ahead or not. Constant progress and a team daring to challenge clinical wisdom keep pushing the boundaries of what is successful.

Too often, the underlying diagnosis is unknown when life or death decisions must be taken, and inevitably some conditions that appear to be reversible will prove irreversible. Plans must be made for the patient, relatives and team to cope with this.

Reversibility

Cardiac failure justifying mechanical support is rarely recoverable solely with medical management. At best, an intervention is required to correct the cause (e.g. coronary revascularization in the case of acute myocardial infarction) or to repair the failed mechanism (e.g. a ruptured papillary muscle).

Recovery is the ideal outcome and will usually be obvious. However, recovery is not the norm, and even a good heart can be impeded by the ECMO support and associated complications.

Veno-arterial ECMO is not conducive to cardiac recovery. Used in the peripheral configuration (see Chapters 3 and 9), it increases the afterload and may lead to overdistension of the left ventricle. Used in the central configuration, it requires opening of the chest to insert and remove the cannulas and is fraught with problems.

Patients with cardiac failure can be bridged to another device, for either the short or long term. Modern short-term devices use the same pump principles as those used for ECMO, the differences being the absence of an oxygenator and the location of the drainage and return cannulas. Short-term ventricular assist devices are easier to manage and lead to fewer complications than ECMO.

Long-term devices are now implanted in the body and are designed to allow patients an independent life.

The return of circulation instituted by the use of ECMO does not always mean full recovery for all organs. Noteworthy is cerebral damage caused by a prolonged period of hypoxia or low flow. Brainstem death is unusual and extensive ischaemic insults are more frequent. Prognostication is difficult. When it is accepted that recovery will not happen, organ donation should be considered.

Specifics considerations

ECMO-assisted cardiopulmonary resuscitation

Sudden cardiac arrest is still a major cause of death in developed countries, despite multiple campaigns to raise awareness of the value of immediate CPR.

The main reasons for poor prognosis in cardiac arrests are a lack of return of spontaneous circulation, re-arrest from haemodynamic instability after the return of spontaneous circulation and hypoxic brain injury. This extremely poor prognosis, especially with refractory cardiac arrest, has led to considering ECMO support as an alternative to conventional CPR. This has been named extracorporeal or ECMO-assisted CPR (eCPR).

The first successful use of eCPR was described by Kennedy in 1966 within a case series of eight patients. The survivor was a 45-year-old woman, who fully recovered after being supported on ECMO following 45 min of CPR. Due to the absence of randomized controlled trials, available data are limited to observational studies and small case series characterized by a large heterogeneity in the age of the patient, the precipitating cause and the duration of CPR before initiation of ECMO.

The resuscitation guidelines of the American Heart Association published in 2010 gave eCPR a class IIb recommendation if the 'no flow' time was brief and the cause of the cardiac arrest was potentially reversible or amenable to heart transplantation or revascularization.

While the importance of a reversible cause is easily understood, the appropriate duration of CPR before ECMO initiation remains unclear. Thus, eCPR was considered after more than 10 min of CPR in two large in-hospital cardiac arrest case series, whereas CPR duration of more than 20 min or even more than 30 min was considered in out-of-hospital cardiac arrest case series.

In 2008, an observational cohort study described the outcome of 135 in-hospital cardiac arrests of cardiac origin and supported with ECMO (Chen *et al.*, 2008a). Overall, 58% of patients were liberated from ECMO and 34% were alive at hospital discharge. Similarly, the same team reported a short- and long-term benefit of eCPR over conventional CPR.

A 3-year prospective observational study compared eCPR for in-hospital patients undergoing CPR for more than 10 min with patients receiving conventional CPR (Chen *et al.*, 2008b). A total of 59 patients were included in the eCPR group after a median of 40 min of CPR. Patients who underwent eCPR had a higher survival rate to discharge and a higher 1-year survival rate. This has also been reported by others, with survival to discharge as high as 41% with an acceptable neurological status in 85% of the patients (Jo *et al.*, 2011).

Interestingly, survival to discharge decreased by about 1% for each 1 min increase in the duration of CPR. The probability of survival was 65, 45 and 19% when the duration of CPR was 10, 30 or 60 min, respectively (Jo *et al.*, 2011).

Details of these and other studies exploring the use of eCPR in hospitals since 2008 are shown in Table 5.4.

This concept has been taken to the out-of-hospital setting, but data from clinical studies are scarce and limited to small case series or case reports, as shown in Table 5.5. Overall survival in these patients is low, with case series reporting between 4 and 36% survival with a favourable neurological outcome noted in 4–27%. Propensity analysis (matching like for like in observational cohorts) has shown that there might be a benefit of using eCPR in this population who are at very high risk of death.

Intractable arrhythmias

Recurrent ventricular fibrillation, ventricular tachycardia and other malignant rhythms are accepted indications for the institution of ECMO.

ECMO will provide adequate support to other organs and allow perfusion of the myocardium if the coronary arteries are patent and the myocardium not distended. Pharmacological or electrical cardioversion are more likely to be successful when the patient is supported with ECMO.

Table 5.4 Main studies in adults on eCPR in in-hospital cardiac arrest patients since 2008

Reference	Study design	Study year	Country	No. of patients	Mean age (years)	Mean CPR duration (min)	No. (%) weaned from ECMO	Hospital discharge survival (survivors/ total no. of patient (%))	Favourable neurological outcome in survivors (number/no. of patients (%))
Chen *et al.* (2008a)	Retrospective	–	Taiwan	135	54	56	79/135 (59%)	46/135 (34%)	NA
Chen *et al.* (2008b)	Prospective	2004–6	Taiwan	59	57	53	29/59 (49%)	17/59 (29%)	9/59 (15%)
Jo *et al.* (2011)	Retrospective	2004–7	South Korea	83	58	37	48/83 (58%)	34/83 (41%)	29/83 (35%)
Shin *et al.* (2011)	Retrospective	2003–9	South Korea	85	60	42	NA	29/85 (34%)	24/85 (28%)
Avalli *et al.* (2012)	Retrospective	2006–11	Italy	24	67	55	14/24 (58%)	11/24 (46%)	9/24 (38%)
Kagawa *et al.* (2012)	Retrospective	2004–11	Japan	61	69	33	36/61 (59%)	22/61 (36%)	20/61 (33%)

NA, not available.

Table 5.5 Main adult studies on eCPR in out-of-hospital cardiac arrest since 2011

Reference	Study design	Study year	Country	Number of patients	Mean age	Mean CPR duration (min)	Weaned from ECMO	Hospital discharge survival (survivor/total patient number) (%)	Favourable neurological outcome in survivors (number/ survivor) (%)
Ferrari et al. (2011)	Retrospective	2007–8	Germany	22	55	49	8/22 (36%)	8/22 (36%)	8/22 (36%)
Mégarbane et al. (2011)	Retrospective	2005–8	France	66	46	155	1/66 (2%)	1/66 (2%)	1/66 (2%)
Le Guen et al. (2011)	Prospective	2008–10	France	51	42	120	2/51 (4%)	2/51 (4%)	2/51 (4%)
Avalli et al. (2012)	Retrospective	2006–11	Italy	18	46	77	3/18 (17%)	1/18 (6%)	1/18 (6%)
Kagawa et al. (2012)	Retrospective	2004–11	Japan	25	56	65	7/25 (28%)	3/25 (12%)	1/25 (4%)
Maekawa et al. (2013)	Prospective	2000–4	Japan	53	54	49	NA	17/53 (32%)	8/53 (15%)

NA, not available

Preventing overdistension of the heart during ECMO is discussed briefly in Chapter 9.

Acute mechanical defect

Patients who present with an acute mechanical defect may be too unwell to survive to surgery. A common example is the patient presenting with an acute papillary muscle rupture during an acute inferior myocardial infarction. Prompt institution of ECMO will allow the patient to receive coronary revascularization in the angiography suite (if appropriate) and then be moved to the operating theatre for the mechanical defect to be fixed.

In these situations, starting ECMO in the peripheral veno-arterial configuration (see Chapter 9) is an immediate life-saving measure. In theatre, the circuit can be converted to a central veno-arterial configuration that can be continued for a few hours or days post-operatively to allow recovery of the stunned heart.

Bridge to heart transplantation or mechanical assist devices

Patients eligible for transplantation or a mechanical device may present with pump failure and organ dysfunction precluding progression to the definitive treatment or support. ECMO will buy time in these conditions, allowing rapid stabilization and optimization of all organs. ECMO is not the best support for the medium to long term, and we advocate using ECMO only for a short period of time. Blood trauma (platelet consumption and overall transfusion requirements) and risk of mechanical complications are greater while on ECMO. The balance of risk to benefit is difficult to gauge and will require discussion between ECMO and transplant physicians and cardiothoracic surgeons. As a rule of thumb, it is surprising when a patient remains on peripheral veno-arterial ECMO for more than 2 weeks without suffering any complications that may be prevented by an early switch to a ventricular assist device. Centre experience in both ECMO and ventricular assistance often influences the decisions. Surgeons may be reluctant to open a chest that is still intact when considering subsequent transplantation and may prefer to prolong the period on veno-arterial ECMO in the hope that a suitable heart may become available. Physicians will be concerned with the recurring transfusion that may increase the titre of human leukocyte antigen (HLA) and other antibodies.

Unable to wean from cardiopulmonary bypass

Patients unable to be weaned from cardiopulmonary bypass are overall poor candidates as they are unlikely to be able to be bridged to a next stage. However, this is not always the case and some may recover (stunned myocardium) or be eligible for transplant or permanent mechanical devices.

The difficulty in these situations is to separate those patients likely to survive from those for whom ECMO will only mean a few more hours or days in intensive care. Clinical judgement is often paramount, and decisions are best made by several clinicians rather than a lone operator. The operating surgeon will invariably be keen to embark on ECMO, subconsciously avoiding a death in the operating room.

If ECMO is considered in such circumstances, it is better to initiate it early rather than inflict multiple insults to the patient's other systems by allowing several episodes of poor perfusion. The institution of ECMO will compound post-operative bleeding, and such patients may end up being stabilized in intensive care with an open chest with surgical packs remaining *in situ* for a few days. A balance between proper haemostasis and thrombus formation needs to be achieved. The most likely location of a thrombus is in the cardiac cavities rather than the ECMO circuit. Anticoagulation will be recommenced at the earliest opportunity. Continuous cardiac ejection should be maintained to prevent blood stasis in the cardiac chambers, as this could cause thrombus formation. Judicious use of inotropes and optimization of ventricular filling are required. Venting of cardiac chambers might be needed to avoid the blood stagnating.

When committed to ECMO, a plan should be agreed and shared with the rest of the team. The patient's next of kin must be prepared for the possibility of failure to recover. Weaning is likely to be difficult (see Chapter 11).

Pulmonary embolism

Pulmonary embolism inspired Gibbon to develop the cardiopulmonary bypass circuit. By maintaining perfusion, allowing gas exchange and avoiding distension of the right ventricle, ECMO was perceived as an ideal tool. This was reinforced by the need to anticoagulant aggressively, an appropriate treatment for pulmonary embolism.

ECMO can still be used in the context of an acute pulmonary embolism that has not resolved. It is, however, an exceptional indication, as many will now be treated by medical therapy (anticoagulation) or less frequently by surgery (Trendelenburg operation).

Successes have been reported in patients suffering from chronic thromboembolic hypertension presenting with superimposed pulmonary embolisms. ECMO can be used in these patients as a bridge to curative operation if their pulmonary disease is amenable to a pulmonary endarterectomy. ECMO can stabilize the patient and allow transportation to a specialist centre.

Other problems requiring cardiopulmonary support

It can be argued that any condition requiring temporary cardiopulmonary support is suitable for ECMO.

ECMO is being used as a mini-cardiopulmonary bypass by some. The main difference with a cardiopulmonary bypass circuit is the absence of a blood reservoir. This has the benefit of removing the blood contact with air, which leads to activation of the inflammatory response. However, it removes the possibility of dissociating drainage from return (allowing the perfusionist to affect the pre- or afterload independently, by specifically adjusting separately the blood drained from or returned to the patient). One disadvantage of using an ECMO circuit as a cardiopulmonary bypass is that air entering the circuit cannot easily be evacuated.

Bridge to organ donation

Starting a patient on ECMO to support the cardiac function ensures optimal perfusion of organs. In the case of irreversible damage to some part of the body leading to survival being impossible, some organs will remain intact for longer. These are then suitable for transplantation.

This is often a very difficult topic for all concerned, but some will find solace when this becomes the outcome of unsuccessful interventions.

ECMO is used by some in deceased patients to maintain organ homeostasis during harvesting. It is used to optimize organ function and render the organs suitable for donation.

Other indications

Accidental hypothermia

Profound accidental hypothermia is a particular case. Survival with no or minor neurological impairment after profound accidental hypothermia is possible even when a number of hours of CPR is required before the initiation of extracorporeal rewarming. Recent guidelines from the International Commission for Mountain Emergency Medicine recommend that in the absence of an alternative cause of death, such as trauma or hypoxia, all patients with hypothermia who do not have vital signs should be considered for CPR. The use of CPR is recommended until extracorporeal rewarming is complete, regardless of the duration of CPR. However, the termination of CPR should be considered when the potassium level is higher than $12\,\text{mmol}\,\text{L}^{-1}$. Neurological recovery from profound hypothermia has been reported after several hours (1–5 h) of eCPR.

Drug intoxication

Because cardiotoxicity induced by a drug overdose could quickly recover after toxic epuration, refractory cardiac arrest and severe shock unresponsive to conventional therapies of poisoned patients may benefit from ECMO. Although data on ECMO use in poisoned patients are scarce, a few case reports have been published, detailing the successful use of ECMO in patients poisoned with various drugs (Table 5.3)

Miscellaneous

Patients presenting with liver failure may go into circulatory shock and support with veno-arterial ECMO has been reported as beneficial in several cases.

Veno-arterial ECMO can help support patients with acute airway obstruction leading to cardiopulmonary instability. Patients with acute bronchial haemorrhage or tracheal tears may need acute resuscitation. Veno-arterial ECMO might be instituted to restore circulation and ventilation, allowing the initial insult to be treated.

When not to use ECMO

ECMO should not be used when there is no treatment available to reverse the current condition. ECMO has inherent risks and patients may end up suffering more as a consequence of the institution of support.

ECMO prediction scores

Physiological scoring systems are developed to assist clinicians in estimating the likely outcome of patients supported with ECMO.

The SAVE (http://www.save-score.com) and RESP (http://www.respscore.com) scores are online calculators that allow calculation of estimated survival. One of the limitations of these scores is the small number of patients used to construct them. These scores do not usually account for those patients considered for ECMO support but declined by experienced clinicians because they are either too well or because ECMO support is considered futile.

Key points

- ECMO provides support and not treatment.
- ECMO can be used in any patient, but not all patients will benefit from ECMO.
- Selection of the right patient is crucial or patients will be harmed and resources wasted.

TO LEARN MORE

Annich GM, Lynch WR, MacLaren G, Wilson JM, Bartlett RH, eds. (2012). *ECMO Extracorporeal Cardiopulmonary Support in Critical Care*, 4th edn. Ann Arbor, MI: Extracorporeal Life Support Organization.

Avalli L, Maggioni E, Formica F, *et al.* (2012). Favourable survival of in-hospital compared to out-of-hospital refractory cardiac arrest patients treated with extracorporeal membrane oxygenation: an Italian tertiary care centre experience. *Resuscitation*, 83, 579–83.

Chen YS, Yu HY, Huang SC, *et al.* (2008a). Extracorporeal membrane oxygenation support can extend the duration of cardiopulmonary resuscitation. *Critical Care Medicine*, 36, 2529–35.

Chen YS, Lin JW, Yu HY, *et al.* (2008b) Cardiopulmonary resuscitation with assisted extracorporeal life-support versus conventional cardiopulmonary resuscitation in adults with in-hospital cardiac arrest: an observational study and propensity analysis. *Lancet*, 372, 554–561.

Ferrari M, Hekmat K, Jung C, *et al.* (2011). Better outcome after cardiopulmonary resuscitation using percutaneous emergency circulatory support in non-coronary patients compared to those with myocardial infarction. *Acute Cardiac Care*, 13, 30–4.

Jo IJ, Shin TG, Sim MS, *et al.* (2011). Outcome of in-hospital adult cardiopulmonary resuscitation assisted with portable auto-priming percutaneous cardiopulmonary support. *International Journal of Cardiology*, 151, 12–7.

Kagawa E, Dote K, Kato M, *et al.* (2012). Should we emergently revascularize occluded coronaries for cardiac arrest? Rapid-response extracorporeal membrane oxygenation and intra-arrest percutaneous coronary intervention. *Circulation*, 126, 1605–13.

Le Guen M, Nicolas-Robin A, Carreira S, *et al.* (2011). Extracorporeal life support following out-of-hospital refractory cardiac arrest. *Critical Care*, 15, R29.

Maekawa K, Tanno K, Hase M, Mori K, Asai Y. (2013). Extracorporeal cardiopulmonary resuscitation for patients with out-of-hospital cardiac arrest of cardiac origin: a propensity-matched study and predictor analysis. *Critical Care Medicine*, 41, 1186–96.

Mégarbane B, Deye N, Aout M, *et al.* (2011). Usefulness of routine laboratory parameters in the decision to treat refractory cardiac arrest with extracorporeal life support. *Resuscitation*, 82, 1154–61.

Peek GJ, Mugford M, Tiruvoipati R, *et al.* Efficacy and
economic assessment of conventional ventilatory support
versus extracorporeal membrane oxygenation for severe
adult respiratory failure (CESAR): a multicentre randomised
controlled trial. *Lancet*, 2009; 374: 1351–63.

Shin TG, Choi JH, Jo IJ, *et al.* (2011). Extracorporeal
cardiopulmonary resuscitation in patients with inhospital
cardiac arrest: a comparison with conventional
cardiopulmonary resuscitation. *Critical Care Medicine*,
39, 1–7.

Chapter 6

Cannulation and decannulation

Introduction

Both the insertion and the removal of ECMO cannulas are key stages of ECMO management. These steps will be referred to as cannulation and decannulation, respectively.

ECMO cannulation must be smoothly done and well planned. Complications can be fatal. Insertion and removal can be supported by checklists, as illustrated in Tables 6.1 and 6.2.

Who should insert the cannula?

Peripheral percutaneous cannulation can be done successfully by any clinician trained in the insertion of a large indwelling cannula.

These clinicians should be trained in using strict aseptic technique. They need to have practised the Seldinger technique on multiple occasions and be organized so that the handling of ECMO needles, guidewires, dilators and cannulas is faultless.

They must have a good knowledge of the vascular (and related) anatomy of all vessels they intend to

Table 6.1 Cannulation insertion checklist

Sign in

Wrist band check and patient confirmed

Red blood cells: 2 units available

Platelets: >100,000 or plan in place

C-arm in place and compatible X-ray table and positioning OK

Time out

Name and role of each person in the room

Procedure explained

Facemasks

Goggles/visors

Lead aprons (if using fluoroscopy)

Cannula size agreed and available

ECMO circuit ready

Back-up plan for failed insertion

Monitoring, including: invasive blood pressure, central venous pressure and end-tidal CO_2

Large venous access secured

Antibiotics

Anticoagulation

Any concerns?

Sign out

Dressing in place

All lines are secured

Instrument count correct

Guidewires and sharps disposed safely

Issues/notes

cannulate. Expertise in ultrasound-guided insertion of vascular lines is a key skill, as this will greatly reduce the incidence of complications. A surprising and deleterious consequence of not using an ultrasound is shown in Figure 6.1.

Table 6.2 Cannulation removal checklist

People

Who is the operator?

Senior clinician and ECMO specialist aware and immediately available

Surgeon present

If surgeon not present, surgeon is immediately available and aware

Scrub nurse or nurse trained in assisting removal of a cannula

Perfusionist present

Identification of roles and responsibilities

Clinical lead clearly stated

Runner identified

Every member aware of what is expected (dry run)

Personal protection for all operators and exposed staff

Gowns for each operator

Goggles for each operator

Facemasks for each operator

Gloves for each operator

Equipment

Dressing pack

Drapes

Stitch cutter

Sutures

Sterile scissors

Specimen pot

Chlorhexidine swabs

Dressing

Procedure

Ensure patient comfortable and sedated if required

Check platelet count and coagulation

Remove dressings, and clean site and cut stitches

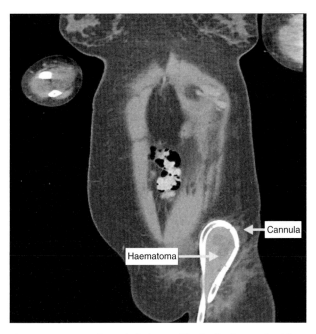

Figure 6.1 A cannula entirely located in the fat in a patient for whom ultrasound was not used to locate the vessel. Surprisingly, the drainage from the haematoma was sufficient to maintain blood flow through the ECMO circuit for at least 1 day.

Clinicians must be aware of the benefits and limitations of using fluoroscopic (X-ray) guidance when inserting a cannula, and be cognisant of the regulations surrounding the use of fluoroscopy in the clinical environment.

While a clinician does not need to be a surgeon to insert an ECMO cannula, vascular and/or cardiothoracic surgeons should be readily available to deal with vascular injuries.

The clinician inserting the ECMO cannula must have the knowledge and skill sets to be able to stabilize a patient having suffered a major vascular injury while surgical input is awaited.

Only trained cardiothoracic surgeons should insert cannulas under direct vision in an open chest.

Where should cannulation take place?

The ideal location to insert the ECMO cannula is in the operating theatre, with the patient positioned on an operating table.

An operating room provides plenty of space. Operating department staff are used to sterile procedures and managing critically ill patients and emergencies. Anaesthetic support allows the clinician inserting the cannula to concentrate on the task at hand, while another highly trained professional ensures that the patient is appropriately managed. It is easier to deal with complications in the operating room, particularly when a surgical intervention is required.

Most operating rooms will provide fluoroscopy (X-ray guidance) if required, and specialist centres will usually have ultrasonography and echocardiography readily available.

Operating rooms upgraded with high-end imaging facilities are ideal; these are hybrid catheter laboratory/operating rooms and are set up to allow complex surgery.

It is possible, but not ideal, to cannulate patients while in their bed or on a trolley, and therefore in any location, including the ICU or emergency room. These locations do not offer the same support. For example, space constraints in the ICU might not permit the use of fluoroscopy. This may be due to lack of shielding and protection of other patients and staff, or the standard catheter laboratory may be inconvenient as the C-arm is not ergonomically positioned to provide full access to the patient's neck.

In the absence of appropriate facilities, the clinician has to weigh up the risk of complications versus the benefits of insertion; this applies mainly for emergency (cardiac arrest) or out-of-hospital insertion. ECMO candidates are usually extremely ill, and many intensive care clinicians claim that these patients are too ill to be transported safely to the operating room. We usually challenge this assumption on the basis of the greater benefit of a safer insertion.

Cannula choice

Main features of a cannula

Cannula choice has to focus on maximizing flow while causing minimal damage to the blood. A generic cannula and some of its features are shown in Figure 6.2.

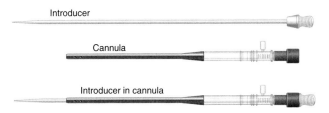

Figure 6.2 An ECMO cannula.

Materials

Flexibility and consistency of shape are influenced by the material of the cannula.

Flexible cannulas are more difficult to insert but can adjust to the patient's anatomy and cause less tissue damage. Too flexible a cannula may kink or collapse, impeding the flow or causing turbulence.

Polyurethane is used in the manufacture of most cannula. It has high material strength at room temperature but is more malleable at body temperature.

Wire reinforcement of the cannula walls will reinforce specific components and prevent kinking or collapse. This enables mobilization of the patient. Radio-opaque materials allow confirmation of correct positioning.

Surface coating

Blood interacting with artificial surfaces activates the coagulation and inflammatory cascades. Coating the surface of the cannula is essential to prevent fibrin sheath and thrombus formation. A small thrombus can have a significant effect on flow.

Modern cannulas feature biocompatible coatings that reduce activation of the clotting cascade. Heparin-coated surfaces are most commonly used and result in reduced inflammatory activation.

Alternatives have been proposed but none yet are as efficient as heparin. However, these are valuable in the context of heparin-induced thrombocytopenia.

Length

The cannula length is often determined by the intended circuit: it is configured short in central access as it is directly in the main vessels or cavities, whereas it is long in a peripheral cannula to reach the intended central location, such as the right atrium for drainage or return.

Shape

The shape of the cannula influences its flow characteristics. Changes in cross-section (tapering), a non-circular cross-section, bends or other irregular shapes can have dramatic effects on flow. There are significant differences between arterial and venous cannulas due to the different physiological requirements.

Venous cannulas need to support high enough drainage flows to sustain adequate support with relatively low negative drainage pressures so that the vessel does not collapse. The collapse of the vena cava with increased drainage suction will hinder drainage. This concept makes the venous cannula diameter the limiting factor for overall flow. The large-capacity veins allow larger-diameter venous cannulas to be inserted. Venous cannulas commonly include side holes to improve drainage.

Arterial cannulas are significantly narrower due to the vessel size, and significantly higher pressures have to be applied for adequate flow. The arterial cannulas provide a large resistance within the ECMO circuit and therefore create a pressure drop across it. This high-pressure flow becomes turbulent at the step-wise increase in flow diameter when exiting the cannula into the artery and forms a jet. This arterial return jet in veno-arterial ECMO can cause a stroke when athero-emboli on the arterial wall are loosened. Potential vessel damage is reduced by specific design of the arterial cannula tip into a 'diffuser tip', where the return jet widens (and therefore slows down), and by the addition of side holes returning blood into the aorta.

Peripheral arterial cannulas are not only significantly longer but also have a smaller diameter throughout, as the peripheral vessel at the insertion point is narrow. Further tapering would only increase the resistance across the cannula.

Generally, cannulas have transitions in shape or material out of necessity – these are usually smooth, but at times steps might be required in the manufacturing process. These steps form targets for turbulence and stagnation, and therefore both hinder flow and predispose to thrombus formation within the cannula.

Side holes

Venous cannulas often have side holes to facilitate better drainage at lower negative pressures. The side holes have been shown to decrease the amount of overall mechanical stress on blood components. They allow greater drainage flow but create local vortices and turbulence. Computational fluid dynamics has been used to evaluate and quantify these effects and has led to improved side-hole placement.

Double lumen

Double-lumen cannulas combine both drainage and return into one cannula. Here, the geometry of the flow and configuration of side holes is complex, as the two flows and the risk of recirculation have to be considered.

Additional features (insertion/side arms)

Cannulas inserted into peripheral arteries may nearly occlude the vessel volume and can cause downstream ischaemia. To avoid this, arterial reperfusion lines should be incorporated into the cannula. These arterial side arms are significantly narrower than the main cannula and therefore have faster flow. The higher chance of turbulence in this setting also raises the likelihood of thrombus formation and blockage of the reperfusion line.

Cannula comparisons

In order to compare different cannulas and determine the best choice for each situation, pressure flow tables are often used. These tables are usually established experimentally and show the behaviour of the cannulas with varying flow speeds.

The advantage of these tables is that the necessary flow can be estimated and the appropriate cannula chosen before insertion. Most tables published in catalogues show the pressure drop corresponding to a flow between 0 and 5 L/min.

In addition to pressure tables, the M-number allows comparison of different cannulas by calculating an effective resistance for each cannula. For example, a practical application to ECMO cannulas showed that the M-numbers for shorter but narrower arterial cannula were identical to those of longer, wider venous ones. As a result, the short and narrow arterial cannulas were preferentially used for percutaneous cannulation.

Selection of the cannula

Many different cannulas are available from a variety of manufacturers.

Cannulas for central veno-arterial ECMO

Cannulas used during surgery can continue to be used to avoid the need for cannula change when central veno-arterial ECMO is established in an emergency. This requires them to perform both for a longer period of time and in different circumstances.

These cannulas are relatively short and have a large diameter, allowing high maximal flow, but increase the risk of dislodgement or movement when used long term.

Electively inserted ECMO cannulas usually have wire-reinforced walls to prevent kinking. The elective arterial cannulas have a smaller diameter, which increases the pressure drop, but has multiple outlet holes that reduce it.

Both bypass and designated ECMO arterial cannulas have diffuser or curved tips to reduce the damage to the arterial vessel wall.

Central veno-arterial ECMO uses two-stage venous cannulas with drainage holes near the tip in the inferior vena cava and an additional drainage 'basket' in the right atrium. This allows a larger diameter along more of the cannula and therefore increased maximal flow. Similarly to the arterial cannulas, the venous cannula walls are reinforced with wire.

One-stage cannulas offer a simpler option; they are easier to insert, but only drain blood from the right atrium.

Cannulas for peripheral veno-arterial ECMO

The vessel size at the insertion site is significantly smaller for an arterial cannula, and the cannula diameter is reduced compared with central ones. This, combined with the increased length, creates a higher pressure drop across the cannula.

A specific feature of peripheral arterial cannulas is the need to add reperfusion lines that aim to prevent leg ischaemia by providing perfusion to the lower limb.

The peripheral venous cannulas are longer than their central counterparts, extending up into the inferior vena cava, and usually have several side holes along their length for improved drainage.

Most of these cannulas have thin wire-reinforced walls to prevent kinking and some are two-stage models that extend into the superior vena cava. The long, extended tip is narrower than the body of the cannula, giving it a tapered shape.

Cannulas for veno-venous ECMO

One of the most recent methods of access for veno-venous ECMO is the use of a double-lumen single cannula, which is inserted into the superior vena cava via the internal jugular vein.

The walls are wire reinforced and have drainage side holes for both the superior vena cava and inferior vena cava.

The return hole needs to be aimed at the tricuspid valve, which requires accurate positioning using fluoroscopy or ultrasound.

One commercially available option for double-lumen cannulas is the Avalon Elite®. It is available in a size range of 13–31 Fr (French scale), with pressure drops of 200 mmHg across the arterial inflow and 60 mmHg across the venous drainage for 4 L/min flow in the 27 Fr cannula.

Another option is the Novaport Twin cannula from Novalung. It is available in three sizes ranging from 18 to 24 Fr with pressure drops of 70 mmHg across the arterial inflow and 30 mmHg across the venous drainage for 2 L/min flow in the 24 Fr cannula.

For single-lumen veno-venous ECMO, normal peripheral venous cannulas are used.

Cannulation technique

The starting point for cannulation should be the identification of the targeted vessel(s) using anatomical landmarks and ultrasound guidance. While most large veins in an adult patient can accommodate a large cannula, measuring the diameters of a target artery (to establish veno-arterial ECMO) can help in selecting the correct cannula size. Some cannulas (i.e. double lumen, drawing from the superior and inferior vena cava and returning in a central position) must always be inserted in the right internal jugular vein. Others can be inserted in any vessel that is large enough.

Aseptic technique should be used throughout. Sterile surgical gowns and gloves should be worn. Facemasks and facial protection protect the staff from blood splashes and must be used.

Two operators are required to insert a cannula, one cannulating and the other assisting. They should have dedicated support to hand them anything required for a smooth insertion.

The needle-to-skin approach should be shallow enough to avoid an abrupt change of angulation at the point of entry in the vein (Figure 6.3).

The location of the needle insertion point has to take into account the subsequent position of the cannula and the potential impact on the patient's mobilization and mobility.

We strongly advocate following the guide-wire progression under fluoroscopy and undertaking repeated

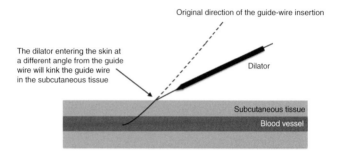

Original direction of the guide-wire insertion

The dilator entering the skin at a different angle from the guide wire will kink the guide wire in the subcutaneous tissue

Dilator

Subcutaneous tissue

Blood vessel

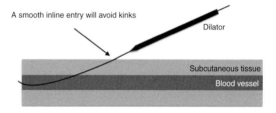

A smooth inline entry will avoid kinks

Dilator

Subcutaneous tissue

Blood vessel

Figure 6.3 Angle of cannulation to avoid a kink in the wires.

checks to ensure that it remains straight and in the correct location. This is, in our view, mandatory if inserting a double-lumen cannula through the jugular vein. Manipulation of the guide wire under fluoroscopy might be required to guide it into the correct location or to avoid looping or the formation of knots.

Dilation of the skin is often required, even with the best-designed cannula. A small skin incision might be required but can cause incessant bleeding after initiation of ECMO, so is best avoided if at all possible.

It is sometimes difficult to know how much force to apply to the cannula during insertion. The absence of movement of the cannula when not caught in skin, muscle or ligament should indicate the need to use a smaller size, as it might be that the vein is too small.

Connection of the cannula to the tubing should ensure that no air is left in the circuit. This requires manual dexterity and coordination between the operator and assistant.

Fixation of the cannula should take as long as, if not longer than, the insertion itself. It should only be done after correct positioning has been confirmed. Correct positioning can only be determined after initiation of ECMO, confirming adequate drainage and return and no obvious recirculation in the case of veno-venous ECMO (see Chapter 4). Fluoroscopy, visual inspection and sometimes ultrasonography will help to achieve this. It is important not to suture the cannula tightly to the skin to prevent skin necrosis and pressure ulcers. Plaster-type fixations can be used successfully in isolation or in combination with standard sutures. Multiple anchorage points are required to prevent inadvertent sudden removal of the cannula.

Reperfusion cannulas

When inserting a veno-arterial ECMO with the return cannula in a peripheral artery (most commonly the femoral), perfusion of the distal part of the vessel must be ensured.

A graft to the side of the vessel could be constructed by a vascular surgeon, allowing blood to flow up and down the vessel. However, this is not always possible due to surgical skill availability. It also entails opening the skin. More importantly, it has been shown to fail on many occasions after several days of support (perhaps due to the high flow immediately at the point of anastomosis).

When the femoral artery has been selected, the best option is to insert a smaller cannula in a distal direction, with the opening of the cannula located below the insertion point of the main cannula (Figure 6.4).

A connection on the return arm of the ECMO circuit is needed to divert some oxygenated blood to this extra line and perfuse the leg. We have found that a single-lumen 6 Fr catheter can be adequate. One tip is to infuse continuously some heparin down that line to avoid occlusion by a thrombus. This side arm can also be used to infuse a vasodilator such as glyceryl trinitrate to ensure homogenous flow distribution. Note that it is easier to insert the reperfusion cannula before inserting the main cannula, and that ultrasound guidance should be used.

Cannula and circuit configuration

While a single double-lumen cannula can be inserted in the right internal jugular vein in the context of veno-venous ECMO, multiple different configurations are possible for all types of ECMO.

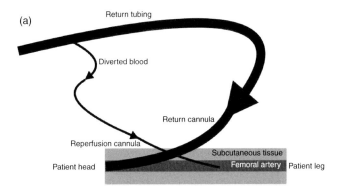

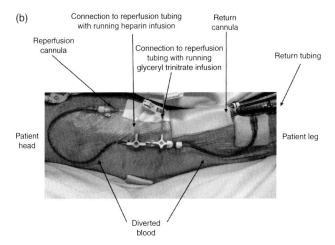

Figure 6.4 (a) Reperfusion cannula inserted in the femoral artery. (b) Reperfusion cannula inserted in the femoral artery, with connection on the reperfusion line with a continuous infusion of heparin.

As a general rule, the drainage cannula should be of greater diameter than the return cannula. Increased drainage can be obtained by inserting another cannula (note: changing a cannula to a larger-diameter one is an exercise few would contemplate: it means interrupting the ECMO circuit while the cannula is exchanged, probably resulting in much blood loss and loss of ECMO support). Note that the flow in each cannula must be high enough at all times to minimize the risk of thrombus formation (see Chapter 3). This can be tricky to achieve when several drainage or return cannulas are in place.

In veno-venous ECMO, the tip of the return cannula should be the closest to the right ventricle, to avoid recirculation (see Chapter 4).

Complications of cannulation

At least 1% of ECMO cannulations will result in major vessel or cardiac perforation. Surgical support must be available or this major risk must be weighed against the benefits of instituting ECMO.

Awareness of the possible complications is required, as standard physiological signs may not be present. Major occult haemorrhage must be expected in the case of sudden haemodynamic deterioration after cannulation. Of note, the end-tidal CO_2 will decrease in all types of ECMO and is not always a sign of tamponade or air embolism (note: it will be a sign if there is a sudden drop before ECMO has been initiated).

Table 6.3 List of possible cannulation complications

Cardiac arrhythmias

Laceration of vascular structure

Haemorrhage, including occult, such as retroperitoneal haematoma, haemothorax and pericardial tamponade

Air embolism

Selective cannulation of smaller vessels, such as azygos, innominate or hepatic veins

Cavitation (bubbles trapped on the cannula wall being released in blood)

Blood trauma, including haemolysis

Compression of other structures (e.g. a venous cannula compressing an artery)

Pneumothorax

After initiation of ECMO, surgical exploration of the insertion point may open one of the cannula side holes to air, leading to massive haemorrhage or air embolism that may surprise a surgeon not used to dealing with ECMO circuits.

Other complications of cannulation are usually well known to the clinicians practised at inserting large indwelling vascular lines and are listed in Table 6.3.

Removal of ECMO cannulas

Removal of a venous cannula

All venous cannulas can be removed using a simple aseptic technique.

This can be done in an awake and cooperative patient and does not require sedation.

A team is required to ensure that resuscitation measures can be established without delay in case of a problem. The operator requires an assistant. The team needs to plan for possible issues. Protective equipment should be used by all team members, as there is a high risk of blood splash on removing a long indwelling cannula.

Patient positioning is crucial to avoid deterioration during the process of removing the cannula. For example, keeping a patient in the supine position for a long period of time may cause distress and ventilatory issues.

The operator must be aware of the risk of air embolism (which could be entrained into the patient's own circulation with devastating consequences), and a positive pressure needs to be applied when the cannula is withdrawn.

The area around the venous cannula should be infiltrated with local anaesthetic and a horizontal mattress suture placed in the cannulation wound (Figure 6.5).

A conscious patient is then asked to perform a Valsalva manoeuvre to prevent air embolism, the tubing is clamped, the cannula is smartly withdrawn by an assistant and the suture is tied. No manual pressure should be applied to the skin, as the lips of the wound will usually close the track and avoid bleeding. Pressure might occlude the vein and lead to the formation of a thrombus.

If the patient is sedated and fully ventilated, positive-pressure ventilation will prevent an air embolism.

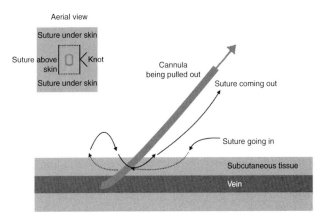

Figure 6.5 A mattress suture.

Note that the vein can be immediately recannulated for a central line (or a new ECMO cannula if it does not go as planned) via a separate skin puncture.

Vein avulsion has been described, and the operator should evaluate a possible cause of cannula retention rather than use brute force.

Removal of a cannula can be supported by a specific checklist, as shown in Table 6.2.

Removal of an arterial cannula

Cannulas inserted surgically should be removed surgically.

Percutaneous arterial cannulas can be removed manually, with subsequent compression of the artery. However, this is not advocated, and surgical removal in the operating room is preferred in all situations.

Care after removal of a cannula

The patient needs to be observed closely. Major haemorrhage remains a possibility.

Key points

- Cannulation should ideally happen in the operating room.
- Ultrasound and fluoroscopy are indispensable adjuncts.
- The benefit of ECMO must outweigh the potential risk of cannulation, even more so if specialist back-up is not readily available.
- Fixation should take as long as insertion and is equally important.

TO LEARN MORE

Annich GM, Lynch WR, MacLaren G, Wilson JM, Bartlett RH, eds. (2012). *ECMO Extracorporeal Cardiopulmonary Support in Critical Care*, 4th edn. Ann Arbor, MI: Extracorporeal Life Support Organization.

Chimot L, Marqué S, Gros A, *et al.* (2013). Avalon bicaval dual-lumen cannula for venovenous extracorporeal membrane oxygenation: survey of cannula use in France. *ASAIO Journal*, 59, 157–61.

Kohler K, Valchanov K, Nias G, Vuylsteke A. (2013). ECMO cannula review. *Perfusion*, 28, 114–24.

Chapter 7

Coagulation, blood and ECMO

Haematology input

Expert haematology support is required when supporting patients on ECMO.

Extracorporeal circulation is only possible if the patient's coagulation is controlled. Exposure of blood to foreign materials triggers the inflammatory response, including the coagulation cascade. Protocols and guidelines for staff must be in place to help manage a fine balance, minimizing both the risk of thrombus formation and that of spontaneous (or aggravated) bleeding.

The blood passing through the circuit will be exposed to different forms of stresses. These will add to the modifications caused by the primary disease or clinical problem leading to the patient requiring support.

Bleeding justifies transfusion of replacement products.

Patients can present with primary haematological disease compounding the complexity of their management.

Most patients will be adequately managed by experienced staff referring to guidelines, but expert advice should always be sought for any deviation.

General considerations

The need for anticoagulation

Most patients supported by ECMO will receive continuous anticoagulation. In some circumstances, the risk of anticoagulation will outweigh its potential benefits.

Heparin-coated circuits allow avoidance of systemic anticoagulation as long as the blood flow is maintained at a high enough rate (probably above 2 L/min) in each component of the circuit. While this seems to be possible for weeks in patients supported with veno-venous ECMO, we would not advocate it in patients requiring veno-arterial ECMO. The changes in flow rheology observed during veno-arterial ECMO may explain why thrombi rapidly develop in blood vessels or cardiac chambers.

Patients supported with ECMO are at risk of dramatic blood loss. These can be iatrogenic (e.g. surgical wound) or spontaneous (e.g. epistaxis or retroperitoneal haemorrhage). Anticoagulant drugs must be easy to titrate and to reverse.

Thrombi formed in a veno-venous circuit that reach the venous circulation will be filtered by the lungs. Thrombi formed in veno-arterial circuits that reach the systemic circulation will have immediate dramatic consequences.

Assays and blood samples

The majority of assays are done using plasma, as whole blood is unstable. The majority of coagulation assays are based on platelet-poor plasma, usually requiring a 10 min centrifugation step. This explains the time-delay between request and result, and the frustration sometimes encountered by the clinical team looking after critically ill patients.

The majority of laboratory analysers are optical instruments. Extreme and sudden changes in the patient's whole-blood composition will impair the laboratory's ability to obtain and interpret valid results. This applies to patients presenting with lipaemia or haemolysis.

To analyse coagulation in particular, mechanical instruments such as the old-fashioned steel ball coagulometer or thromboelastograph can get results where optical instruments will fail.

Frequent blood sampling is a significant source of iatrogenic anaemia. Intelligent scheduling and the use of smaller quantities (such as used in paediatric patients) may help to alleviate this issue.

Choice of anticoagulant

The ideal anticoagulant for patients on ECMO would be highly effective in reducing thrombotic events; carry a low rate of bleeding events; exhibit a rapid and predictable dose response in a variety of clinical scenarios; have easy, cheap and accurate point-of-care monitoring; and have no drug interactions.

Unfractionated heparin

Unfractionated heparin remains the mainstay of continuous anticoagulation therapy in the patient on ECMO support due to its rapid onset of action and the ability to reverse its action with protamine. It is used daily in thousands of patients.

When given intravenously, the heparin half-life is short (30–90 min depending on dose). The onset is immediate when given as a bolus. Heparin can be used to form an inner anticoagulant surface on various devices, such as ECMO tubing, cannulas and oxygenator components.

Pharmacological heparin is a complex bioextract obtained from bovine lung or porcine intestine. The anticoagulant activity per unit of heparin varies among manufacturers, as does its reversibility by protamine in U/mg.

Heparin action is dependent on the presence of functional antithrombin in the patient and acts on the clotting factors IIa, Xa, IXa and XIa. The avidity to these factors will vary depending on the unfractionated heparin chain length and sulfation.

Elimination is both by poorly characterized internal absorption pathways (through macrophages, platelets and endothelium) and renally. Clinically significant half-life prolongations are not observed in renal failure.

The optimal dose of heparin sufficient to prevent thrombosis without causing bleeding is not known.

Fractionated heparin and pentasaccharides

Drugs such as low-molecular-weight heparin (LMWH) and fondaparinux are not used routinely in patients supported with ECMO as they cannot easily be reversed and have long half-lives in some circumstances. New antidotes are being developed and may allow the safe use of agents other than heparin in patients supported with ECMO.

Fractionated heparin or LMWH are the result of breaking down polymeric heparin salts into smaller components. Their effect is easier to predict than those of unfractionated heparin. Their action is dependent on antithrombin. Despite being a shorter version of heparin, LMWH has a long half-life and is excreted exclusively by the kidneys. The reversibility varies, and LMWH can be partially reversed by protamine. This is more effective shortly after the LMWH has been administered but cannot entirely be predicted, so is impractical.

Fondaparinux is a pentasaccharide and its action is antithrombin dependent. Fondaparinux cannot be reversed with protamine and has a very long half-life (17 h). It is excreted by the kidneys.

Direct thrombin inhibitors

Intravenous direct thrombin inhibitors are available. Those used in patients supported with ECMO have short half-lives and cannot be reversed. Their use is often limited to patients with heparin-induced thrombocytopenia.

Monitoring of anticoagulation

The effect of anticoagulants has to be monitored closely to achieve the best balance between avoidance of thrombus

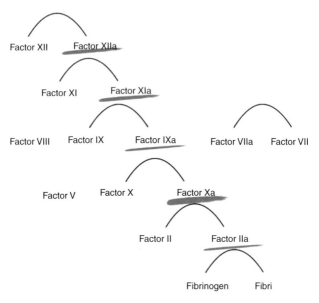

Figure 7.1 Clotting cascade. The relative inhibitory effect of heparin on various steps is indicated by highlighting, together with the relative position of factor Xa in the coagulation cascade.

formation and risk of bleeding. This can usually be achieved with heparin levels between 0.3 and 1.0 U/mL. Of note, this is around five times lower than the concentration obtained during cardiac surgery with cardiopulmonary bypass (during which the blood is subjected to surgical trauma and exposed to air).

Heparin acts at various levels of the coagulation cascade, as shown in Figure 7.1.

Heparin monitoring

There is no calibrated reference standard, as seen for anticoagulation with vitamin K inhibitors for which the international normalized ratio (INR) is used. The anti-factor Xa (anti-Xa) level is the closest reference standard available.

Activated coagulation time

The activated coagulation time (ACT) was devised by Hattersley in 1966 for the care of patients with severe haemophilia requiring heparin monitoring. The ACT records the time between exposure in a tube of whole blood to glass (contact activation) and the formation of a visible thrombus.

The ACT is sensitive to heparin and measures the heparin effect rather than the level. Factors beyond the plasma coagulation affect the absolute result, as it is a whole-blood assay.

There is no universally agreed therapeutic range. It is a near-patient assay. Most hospitals have not validated their in-house ACT cartridges and do not know how this value correlates with their coagulation tests (which are highly variable from institution to institution). Each hospital should validate the ACT measurements to either their laboratory activated prothrombin time (aPTT) or anti-Xa measures to ensure that the adopted ACT range is at least comparable to the laboratory coagulation tests range. An example is shown in Figure 7.2. The ACT tests will vary in their sensitivity to heparin, and different systems should be used to monitor various clinical settings (e.g. an ACT system designed to be used during

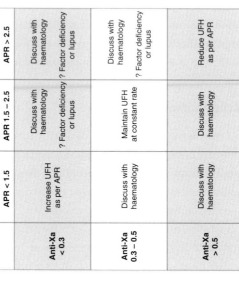

	APR < 1.5	APR 1.5 – 2.5	APR > 2.5
Anti-Xa < 0.3	Increase UFH as per APR	Discuss with haematology ? Factor deficiency or lupus	Discuss with haematology ? Factor deficiency or lupus
Anti-Xa 0.3 – 0.5	Discuss with haematology	Maintain UFH at constant rate	Discuss with haematology ? Factor deficiency or lupus
Anti-Xa > 0.5	Discuss with haematology	Discuss with haematology	Reduce UFH as per APR

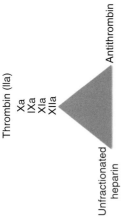

Thrombin (IIa)

Xa
IXa
XIa
XIIa

Unfractionated heparin

Antithrombin

Figure 7.2 Relationship between anti-Xa and ACT, as well as the interrelationship between anti-thrombin, unfractionated heparin and thrombin. APR, activated prothrombin time ratio; UFH, unfractionated heparin.

cardiac surgery will monitor much higher doses of heparin than systems used during ECMO).

Activated prothrombin time

The aPTT is triggered by exposing platelet-poor plasma to phospholipids and sand. Centrifugation from whole blood to platelet-poor plasma introduces a delay of 10 min in obtaining a result. Using platelet-poor plasma introduces a bias that is dependent on the composition of the patient's whole blood when trying to compare it directly with the ACT. The aPTT is relatively inexpensive.

The aPTT measures the heparin effect rather than the heparin level. It can be validated against heparin protamine titration by performing the test repeatedly with increasing doses of protamine added to neutralize the heparin effect in the sample.

The activated prothrombin time ratio (APR) is a modification of the aPTT result: the patient's aPTT (measured in seconds) is divided by the mean of the normal range (in seconds). The APR is a dimensionless ratio (e.g. 1.5) but must not be confused with the INR. The aPTT range and APR must be standardized to heparin protamine titration in each laboratory, as it is dependent on the reagent providers or analysers.

The sensitivity of the test varies between different reagent manufacturers. Care must be taken when adopting the aPTT ranges validated in another centre, as this may use a different aPTT/analyser combination.

The aPTT will also be affected by the presence of lupus anticoagulant, or by changes in factor VIII, IX, XI and XII levels.

Anti-Xa levels

The anti-Xa level has replaced heparin protamine titration as the 'gold standard' test for some of the fractionated heparins.

The anti-Xa level can measure heparin effect (if patient endogenous antithrombin is used in the assay) or heparin level (if exogenous antithrombin is added to the assay). The ECMO physician should establish whether the assay uses exogenous antithrombin or not, as this will affect interpretation of the results.

The anti-Xa level measurement is performed in platelet-poor plasma and therefore is not comparable to the whole-blood ACT. The anti-Xa level does not measure the inhibition of factors XIa, IXa and IIa, and will only reflect part of the unfractionated heparin activity.

The anti-XA level will only be slightly affected by global changes in coagulability, such as that observed in disseminated intravascular coagulation.

The anti-Xa level requires initial calibration by the laboratory but can then be compared between different centres. In ECMO support, a multicentre consensus appears to be obtaining anti-Xa levels of 0.3–0.5 IU/mL. These are lower than the levels required when treating venous thrombosis (0.5–1.0 IU/mL).

Thromboelastography

Thromboelastography is a functional test that measures the viscoelastic properties of blood and evaluates the whole clotting system, including platelet function, clotting factors and fibrinolysis.

The use of thromboelastography during ECMO can sometimes be useful in bleeding patients, but it will not detect some antiplatelet effects (it will usually be normal in patients on aspirin). The addition of various reagents such as heparinase facilitates the interpretation of thromboelastography.

How important are all these tests?

Specialist input will save lives, but this is not always obvious to the bedside clinician.

This can be shown in the example of a patient admitted with acute heart failure following CPR and established on ECMO. A first dose of heparin was administered on cannulation and an aPTT obtained several hours later showed an APR of 4.8. The heparin dose was progressively decreased and the APR levelled at 1.9. Despite what was thought adequate anticoagulation, multiple thrombi developed in the cardiac chambers. Anti-Xa levels were found to be disproportionally low in relation to APR, and further testing revealed a deficiency in factor XI. Multimodal monitoring would have detected this anomaly earlier.

Standard decision trees should be developed to support staff at the bedside. This should include when to call the haematology department (see example in Figure 7.3).

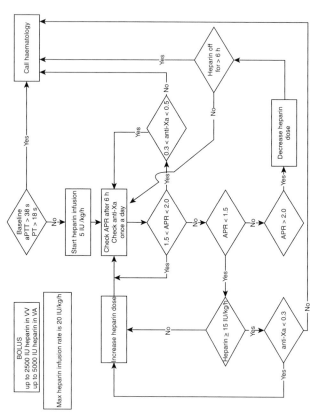

Figure 7.3 Example of a decision tree to support staff at the bedside. VA, veno-arterial; VV, veno-venous; PT, prothrombin time.

Blood product transfusion

Major blood losses can happen in patients supported by ECMO, and provision of compatible units of blood and blood products should be immediately available.

Some patients may receive repeated transfusions, and up to 4% of them will develop red blood cell antibodies. This means that compatibility tests should be repeated, usually every 72 h. The presence of antibodies requires repeated cross-matching of the patient's serum to detect the emergence of additional antibodies.

Women of child-bearing age who are rhesus negative must be given special attention, and haematology should always be involved to decide whether it is justified to give anti-D serum.

Abnormalities of blood count

Thrombocytopenia

A large number of critically ill patients experience thrombocytopenia. A very severe numerical thrombocytopenia may show only minimal bleeding. Thrombocytopenia can be caused by reduced production or increased destruction of platelets.

Platelets are produced in response to thrombopoietin secreted by the liver. Platelets can vary considerably in size. Generally, large platelets are more active than small platelets, and are more efficient in thrombus formation.

The main treatment for thrombocytopenia is platelet transfusion. The majority of thrombocytopenic patients recover their platelet count when ECMO is discontinued.

Clinicians' opinion on the minimum platelet threshold that is safe is very variable and ranges from a platelet count of 20×10^9 to 150×10^9. This difference is not confined to the field of ECMO.

Clinicians should measure the increment of a platelet transfusion. A satisfactory platelet increment is an increase by at least 10×10^9/L measured 60 min after infusion. Inconsistent increments between platelet transfusions may alert the clinician to HLA immunization.

Platelets have minimal ABO-system antigen expression but express HLA class I antigens. The HLA class I antigens can immunize the patients and cause refractoriness to certain donors but not others. It is possible to source HLA-matched platelets.

Immunization of HLA can occur in pregnancy or through red blood cell transfusion, and therefore can be observed in all patients, even if never exposed to platelet transfusion.

Heparin-induced thrombocytopenia

Heparin-induced thrombocytopenia (HIT) is a rare complication of using heparin and can be seen in ECMO patients. It is caused by antibodies that are also frequently found in patients exposed to unfractionated heparin during ECMO support. Only a minority of patients will have platelet-activating antibodies.

The diagnosis remains a clinical diagnosis. A laboratory test has a high negative-predictive value (so it is very unlikely to be

HIT even if you thought it was) but a low positive-predictive value (so it is unlikely to be HIT if you thought it was not). Confirmatory methods require great expertise and are only available in selected centres, which causes major delays.

Most of the equipment in common use in ECMO is heparin coated. Heparin-free ECMO is a major challenge and may not be possible for the patient who has been diagnosed with HIT.

Outcomes vary, and generally the prognosis of HIT on ECMO is poor unless ECMO can be discontinued and heparin-free anticoagulation commenced. Heparin-coated material and *in situ* platelet transfusion should be kept to a minimum and only be considered in life-threatening situations after the systemic administration of heparin has been discontinued. Removal of the heparin-coated material is the only solution and this will allow the reaction to subside. Alternative anticoagulation can then be instituted, but haematology expert advice must be sought as there is a greater risk of coagulation imbalance leading to thrombosis.

Anticoagulation of a patient on ECMO with anticoagulant other than heparin is possible. The main challenge is the irreversible nature of the anticoagulant.

Other causes of thrombocytopenia

The cause of thrombocytopenias in the ECMO patient often cannot be identified, but some can be treated, so it is always worthwhile seeking specialist advice.

Acute or 'acute on chronic' immune thrombocytopenia justifies the administration of prednisolone and intravenous immunoglobulin. Immunoglobulins may sometimes be useful to contain thrombocytopenia observed after transfusion or transplant, which is often markedly more haemorrhagic than immune thrombocytopenia.

Drug-induced thrombocytopenia can be profound and should be excluded.

Thrombocytopenia can be related to the primary insult, justifying the use of ECMO. Thrombotic thrombocytopenia purpura is rare and is characterized by fever, intravascular microangiopathic haemolysis, thrombocytopenia, and renal and central nervous system symptoms caused by hyaline thrombi in the brain and kidney (but not in the lungs). Sepsis and haemophagocytic syndrome may present with extremes of pancytopenia.

A bone marrow biopsy may be helpful, particularly in patients presenting with thrombocytopenia. This can be performed safely on a thrombocytopenic patient, even if supported with ECMO.

Arbitrary transfusion thresholds are often unachievable in patients with multifactorial platelet consumption. Empirical approaches can be adopted, such as platelet transfusions every 12 h and intravenous administration of immunoglobulins or use of HLA class I-matched platelets, even in the presence of a negative antibody screen.

Other changes in the blood film

The haematologist will see multiple changes on the blood films. One such example is shown in Figure 7.4.

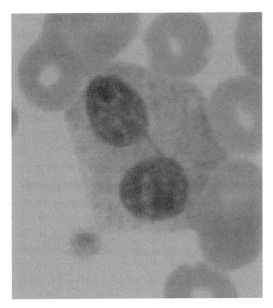

Figure 7.4 The 'sign of dreadfulness': pseudo-pelgerization of neutrophils and prominent basophilic inclusion bodies in the red blood cells show acanthocytosis suggesting hepatic failure, and a nucleated red blood cell is seen adjacent to a mature neutrophil.

Neutrophilia, monocytosis and lymphopenia are common findings, especially during acute exacerbations of septic episodes. The white cells are often affected by the drugs being administered.

Haemolysis

Intravascular or extracorporeal haemolysis is a frequent complication of ECMO.

Haemolysis can be monitored by examining the blood film and measuring lactic dehydrogenase, haptoglobin and plasma-free haemoglobin. High levels of free haemoglobin can interfere with the optical instruments used in the laboratory to measure enzyme levels or coagulation tests.

Significant haemolysis may lead to anaemia followed by inappropriate investigations if not readily recognized.

Severe intravascular haemolysis should be investigated, and causes other than ECMO should be suspected.

ECMO-related haemolysis can be decreased by appropriate circuit management and aiming for the lowest possible blood flow. Multiple thrombosis in the circuit can lead to haemolysis, and replacement of the oxygenator can be a simple solution. Folic acid supplementation may alleviate symptoms.

Haemoglobinopathy patients

Special care has to be taken in the care of haemoglobinopathy patients. They should only be transfused with Rh- and Kell-matched blood products, and the full genotype match for Rh should be obtained to decrease the risk of antibody formation.

Sickle cell patients should, in addition, only be transfused sickle cell haemoglobin (HbS)-negative blood. About 10% of sickle cell patients may require cover with intravenous immunoglobulins and/or steroids if previously declared not transfusable. Frequent exchange transfusion to maintain the HbS level at less than 30% while critically ill is possible in sickle cell patients supported on ECMO.

Bleeding in patients on ECMO

Bleeding is an important cause of morbidity and mortality in patients on ECMO.

Minor bleeding (e.g. at the site of the cannula, line insertions or chest drains) is common in patients on ECMO. Minor bleeding often does not require any intervention other than local pressure. Persistent 'minor' bleeding (e.g. from a neck line suture) may result in significant volume loss if left unchecked for many hours and should not be left untreated.

External visible bleeding (e.g. from the site of a chest drain) should prompt assessment for occult bleeding (e.g. into the pleural space).

Major bleeding is a less common but serious complication. Gastrointestinal bleeding occurs in 5% and pulmonary haemorrhage in 10% of adults receiving ECMO support for respiratory failure.

Intracranial haemorrhage occurs in less than 5% of patients but is a feared complication of ECMO. Neurosurgical consultation is advised and, while most cases are not amenable to surgical correction, it should not be considered a reason to end support with ECMO. Veno-venous ECMO can be continued for weeks without any other anticoagulant than the heparin coating on the circuit, and some patients fully recover.

Measures to prevent bleeding include close attention to anticoagulation and judicious administration of blood products. Avoidance of any unnecessary surgical procedures is the most important way to prevent bleeding.

Any invasive procedures, whether in the operating theatre (e.g. thoracotomy) or at the bedside (e.g. vascular access, chest drain insertion, tracheostomy), including seemingly 'minor' procedures (e.g. nasogastric tube insertion, transoesophageal echocardiography), can all be the cause of significant bleeding.

Lumbar puncture is contraindicated. Intramuscular injections and venepuncture for blood sampling should be avoided

Management of bleeding in patients on ECMO involves optimization of coagulation using blood products, administration of drugs and surgical correction of the cause of bleeding. A suggested outline is given in Table 7.1.

The first step is to rapidly assess the degree of haemorrhage. Major bleeding with haemodynamic compromise should prompt urgent intravascular volume resuscitation, ideally with cross-matched blood, and may require early surgical intervention.

Continued bleeding, despite optimization of platelet count, coagulation parameters and corrective surgery where indicated, should prompt further haematological input.

There is little trial evidence for the use of specific drug therapy in the management of bleeding in patients on ECMO, and support for particular agents is based on anecdotal reports.

Lysine analogues such as tranexamic acid and aminocaproic acid can prove useful in cases of fibrinolysis. Fibrinolysis that occurs suddenly in a patient on ECMO can sometimes be corrected by changing the oxygenator. The most likely reason is the build-up of small thrombi in the oxygenator fibres leading to continuous activation of fibrinolysis.

Table 7.1 Management of bleeding in patients on ECMO involving optimization of coagulation using blood products, administration of drugs and surgical correction of the cause of bleeding

Minor bleeding only

Local measures for superficial minor bleeding: apply pressure, packing

Ongoing 'minor' bleeding

Manage as above

Correction of clotting abnormalities: optimize platelet count (>150,000 using platelet transfusion), INR (<1.5 by transfusion of fresh frozen plasma), fibrinogen (>2.0 using cryoprecipitate)

Consider lower target for heparinization (e.g. lower ACT, aPTT or heparin level range). Maintain circuit flow above 1–2 L/min to reduce risk of thrombosis

Major bleeding

Manage as above

Simultaneous intravascular volume resuscitation, correction of clotting abnormalities and consideration of surgery

Consider infusion of aprotinin

Surgical intervention if probable remediable cause, bleeding is severe or large haematoma

Decrease heparin to low dose (e.g. 5–10 U/kg/h) or no heparin

Haematological specialist advice: consider further tests (e.g. platelet function tests)

Consider separation from ECMO earlier than planned to remove need for heparin and stimulus for further bleeding

Consider administration of clotting factor concentrates if ECMO continuation necessary (associated with a high risk of circuit clotting)

Administration of recombinant factor VIIa is possible but may be associated with higher morbidity, as seen in patients undergoing cardiothoracic surgery.

Surgical intervention may be necessary to remove large haematomas acting as a continued trigger for fibrinolysis. Surgery should be carried out by an appropriately experienced practitioner, with meticulous attention to haemostasis. In difficult-to-control bleeding, packing followed by a scheduled return to theatre may be necessary, allowing time for correction of clotting abnormalities, hypothermia and acidosis.

Key points

- Heparin is the main anticoagulant used in ECMO patients.
- The optimal dose of heparin is unknown.
- A combination of haematological tests should be used in ECMO patients, and the haematologist consulted on many occasions.

TO LEARN MORE

Murphy DA, Hockings LE, Andrews RK, *et al.* (2015). Extracorporeal membrane oxygenation-hemostatic complications. *Transfusion Medicine Reviews*, 29, 90–101

Chapter 8

Management of the patient on veno-venous ECMO: general principles

Introduction

Veno-venous ECMO allows gas exchange and is used to support failing lungs. The cardiovascular system remains intact, and the heart continues to pump the blood around the patient's body.

A simplified view of veno-venous ECMO is that the blood is taken from and returned to the venous system. If the blood is circulated through a functioning oxygenator, gas exchange will happen. If there is no oxygenator (or no gas flow through the oxygenator), the blood will just return in the same state as it drained (perhaps a bit cooler if no heat exchanger is in place). The whole-blood volume (including the proportion that went through the ECMO circuit) is pumped by the heart through the lungs and circulation.

Veno-venous ECMO is usually instituted in the context of severe acute respiratory failure. It supports oxygenation and CO_2 removal and allows the implementation of safer ventilation strategies. This is inaccurately referred to as 'protective' ventilation (any positive-pressure ventilation is deemed to cause damage to the lung) and could be called the 'least-damaging lung ventilation'.

Veno-venous ECMO can be continued for as long as appropriate; investigations are directed at confirming the underlying diagnosis and ensuring specific therapy is administered.

Patients supported with veno-venous ECMO frequently have additional non-pulmonary organ failure and require a high level of critical care support (e.g. acute renal failure).

The day-to-day management of patients on veno-venous ECMO includes all that is common to critically ill patients plus some specific elements. This chapter describes those specific elements.

Locally agreed protocols for the care of ECMO patients should be incorporated into training.

Monitoring of the patient on veno-venous ECMO has been described in Chapter 4.

Stabilization on veno-venous ECMO

Insertion of ECMO cannulas should ideally take place in an operating room. A variety of configurations can be used. It is often striking how rapidly ventilation and other support can be modified after veno-venous ECMO support has been started.

Lung ventilation can be adapted immediately after veno-venous ECMO has been established. The aim is to institute a less-damaging mechanical ventilation with lower levels of pressure. Multiple publications are available, but most clinicians would agree to aim for a standard setting (Table 8.1). Veno-venous ECMO circuits are very efficient at

Table 8.1 Example of standard ventilation settings while on veno-venous ECMO

Peak airway pressure <25 cmH$_2$O (strictly less than 30 cmH$_2$O)

Tidal volume ≤ 6 mL/kg

Positive end-expiratory pressure (PEEP) at 10 cmH$_2$0

Respiratory rate at 10 min

FiO$_2$ 30–50%

Inspiratory : expiratory ratio of 1 : 2

Allow spontaneous breaths within pressure and volume parameters

exchanging CO$_2$. While unproven, it makes sense to decrease the patient PaCO$_2$ progressively to avoid extreme vasoactive responses. This can easily be achieved by initiating veno-venous ECMO with a low gas sweep through the oxygenator (e..g 2 L/min) that is progressively increased (e.g. within the first hour). A low gas sweep will usually not affect oxygenation as transfer of O$_2$ will be limited by other factors (as long as the delivered fraction of O$_2$ in the sweep gas is 100%). In veno-venous ECMO, the inspired fraction of O$_2$ in the sweep gas should always be 100%. As explained in previous chapters, oxygenation in patients supported with veno-venous ECMO is dependent on the blood flow in the circuit in relation to the patient's cardiac output.

Inotropes and other vasoactive drugs will often have been increased to very high levels to maintain some haemodynamic stability in critically ill patients awaiting veno-venous ECMO (often wrongly interpreted as a reason to consider veno-arterial support). This is often exacerbated by high airway and intrathoracic pressure, low O$_2$ levels, high doses of sedative agents, high CO_2 and profound acidosis. The rate of infusion of these drugs can (and should) very often be decreased rapidly.

Red blood cell transfusion is advocated by some, as the O_2 content in the blood will be limited and extra red blood cells will increase the O_2-carrying capacity. Others advocate the use of restrictive transfusion policies identical to those used in other critically ill patients. Justification for a liberal transfusion strategy is that veno-venous ECMO rarely increases the PaO_2 to normal physiological levels. In the absence of a guarantee that a PaO_2 as low as 6 kPa is acceptable, many clinicians will transfuse in the early stages of support. The increased oncotic pressure offered by red blood cell transfusion may be added benefit in critically ill patients in whom the systemic inflammatory response is increased by the use of an ECMO circuit.

If the PaO_2 remains low despite optimal blood flow through the ECMO circuit, it can be presumed that the issue is either inadequate flow for body weight (especially in patients in excess of 100 kg) or high cardiac output leading to a small proportion of circulating blood going through the ECMO circuit. Solutions to this problem include: (1) the insertion of an additional drainage cannula to increase flow through the ECMO circuit as long as the return cannula can accommodate the increase in flow and pressure; and (2) measures to decrease O_2 consumption (such as cooling the core temperature using the heater/cooler in the ECMO circuit to modify the patient's body temperature) or actions to reduce the cardiac output (β-blockers are sometimes used to achieve this, but questions remain on the overall physiological impact this may have). (Note that double-lumen cannulas have an optimized return lumen size for the drainage lumen size, and that adding an extra cannula to improve flow will have only a limited effect.)

If the venous blood is highly desaturated, a second oxygenator may be incorporated into the circuit. While this is difficult to model, this definitely increases the transit time for blood in each oxygenator, and post-oxygenator PaO_2 will be higher.

After stabilization, the patient can now undergo multiple non-invasive tests to determine the cause and remedy the insult that led to respiratory failure.

Oxygenation during veno-venous ECMO

During veno-venous ECMO support, fully O_2-saturated blood from the ECMO circuit mixes in the right atrium with deoxygenated venous return that has not passed through the ECMO circuit, and then passes into the right ventricle and pulmonary artery.

Systemic arterial oxygenation is determined by the relative proportions of oxygenated ECMO blood flow and deoxygenated venous return, and by the degree of pulmonary dysfunction, O_2 consumption, amount of recirculation in the ECMO circuit and oxygenator efficiency.

As described in Chapter 4, recirculation refers to oxygenated blood from the return cannula flowing directly to the drainage cannula of the ECMO circuit, without passing through the lungs and systemic circulation. Recirculation can be identified by high O_2 saturation in the drainage limb (pre-oxygenator) of the ECMO circuit, and often by visual inspection of the drainage limb for 'flashes' of red oxygenated blood mixing with deoxygenated blood. The recirculation fraction increases with increasing ECMO flow. At higher ECMO flow rates, the beneficial effect of increasing flow on the proportion of oxygenated blood entering the pulmonary artery will be offset by an increase in recirculation. In these circumstances, reducing pump speed may actually result in improved oxygenation. Recirculation is higher with a suboptimally positioned ECMO cannula (the best distance between the tip of two cannulas is said to be 10 cm), low cardiac output and low intravascular (specifically right atrial) volume.

ECMO blood flow should initially be set to deliver the maximum flow, typically 5 L/min, without excessive negative pressure in the drainage limb of the ECMO circuit; this should produce a rise in arterial O_2 saturation. Sweep gas should be kept at 100% O_2. Thereafter, oxygenation can be controlled by adjusting circuit blood flow and not by altering FiO_2 or positive end-expiratory pressure (PEEP) on the ventilator. Generally a PaO_2 greater than 6 kPa (50 mmHg) and O_2 saturation greater than 85% are adequate. Occasionally, lower values have to be accepted.

Hypoxaemia while on veno-venous ECMO should be assessed and managed as outlined in Table 8.2.

Table 8.2 Assessment and management of hypoxaemia during veno-venous ECMO

Problem	Causes
Reduction or loss of circuit flow	Low intravascular volume, kink in circuit tubing, obstruction from large thrombus in circuit/oxygenator/cannula, cannula malposition, cardiac tamponade, tension pneumothorax
Post-oxygenator blood not fully saturated	Failing oxygenator, accidental interruption of sweep gas supply
Increased recirculation	ECMO circuit flow too high, suboptimally positioned ECMO cannula, low cardiac output, low intravascular volume
Increase in cardiac output	Sepsis, inotropic drug therapy
Increase in O_2 consumption	Inadequate sedation, seizures, fever
New or worsening lung problem	Malpositioned endotracheal tube (bronchial position or accidental extubation), pneumothorax, segmental lung collapse, worsening consolidation, pulmonary oedema, haemothorax, pulmonary haemorrhage

Management

Treat underlying cause (see above)

Ensure sweep gas is 100% oxygen

Increase ECMO flow; if recirculation is suspected, decreasing ECMO flow may improve systemic oxygenation

Increase FiO_2 on ventilator temporarily

Consider adjuncts such as prone positioning, inhaled nitric oxide

Reduce O_2 consumption by cooling and/or paralysis

Consider additional ECMO cannula if adequate ECMO flow not achieved despite optimization of preload and cannula position

Accept lower targets (e.g. partial pressure of oxygen (paO_2) 6 kPa, saturations 85%) in exceptional circumstances

Consider transfusion of haemoglobin to higher target to increase O_2 delivery

Consider adding second oxygenator

Mechanical ventilation in patients during veno-venous ECMO

Decreasing the impact of mechanical ventilation is thought to be one of the reasons that veno-venous ECMO is of benefit in patients with acute lung injuries.

Ventilator-associated lung injury can be limited by reducing the tidal volume and airway pressures. As the gas exchange is almost fully supported by ECMO, a reduction in mechanical ventilation will allow less-damaging ventilation, so-called 'protective' ventilation. Most patients can be managed with tidal volumes lower than 6 mL/kg of predicted body weight and peak airway pressures lower than 25 cmH$_2$O.

It is possible to stop all mechanical ventilation. In some scenarios, this is the only option available (e.g. massive lung haemorrhage). It is unknown whether the absence of ventilation is better than a low level of mechanical ventilation.

Selected patients can be woken up during veno-venous ECMO, extubated and left to breathe spontaneously. (The respiratory drive can be decreased or even stopped by adjusting the level of gas sweep across the oxygenator. Some patients may be awake and talking but not ventilating.)

High-frequency oscillatory ventilation is an alternative approach to providing 'protective' ventilation, and may be useful in combination with ECMO in patients with severe barotrauma. In these situations, ultra lung rest may be provided by using high-frequency oscillatory ventilation with a low mean airway pressure.

Tidal volume and peak inspiratory pressure

An ideal tidal volume of 6 mL/kg is merely an arbitrary volume chosen by the Acute Respiratory Distress Syndrome Clinical Network (ARDSNet) investigators and shown to be better than a higher volume. In fact, sick lungs may not be able to accommodate a tidal volume of 6 mL/kg.

Selecting a maximum peak pressure is an added safety measure, as the plateau pressure will be lower. Ideally, the chosen pressure should be below the upper inflection point on a pressure–volume curve (after which the pressure rises rapidly with no increase in volume).

The transthoracic pressure is theoretically more important, and multiple measures can be taken. In practical terms, limiting the peak airway pressure to a maximum of 30 cmH_2O seems to be right. Most patients can be managed with peak airway pressures lower than 25 cmH_2O.

Positive end-expiratory pressure

The best PEEP is the one that avoids alveolar collapse and lowers wall stress on inflation. It should not affect the patient's haemodynamic status to a great extent.

The pressure–volume curve can be helpful, as the opening pressure can be seen as the lung starts to inflate, but its interpretation can be complex and it needs to account for lung hysteresis. Moreover, this is compounded by the fact that the lung, even more so when diseased, is not homogenous.

Patients with bronchospasm may trap some air, building their own PEEP.

Mode of ventilation

Pressure control modes are the most logical modes of ventilation in patients with lung injury. Alternatively, volume control modes with a strict limit in the set peak pressures allow a reduction of the damaging effects of mechanical lung ventilation.

Spontaneous modes can be used in awake patients. Of note, awake patients with severe lung injury will often appear distressed because they are tachypnoeic. Tachypnoea is not always a sign of distress, as a small lung vital capacity will lead to an earlier triggering of stretch receptors, leading to a compensatory high respiratory rate.

Adjuncts to mechanical ventilation

Fluid balance

Removing excess water optimizes lung mechanics and pulmonary gas exchange. This should be initiated as soon as possible after veno-venous ECMO initiation.

Removing excess water may be difficult in the first few hours of ECMO support because of the acute response caused by the primary insult and the intense inflammatory response caused by the ECMO circuit. It is, however, critical to ensure that this happens as soon as the acute inflammatory response is controlled and stability has been established.

Tracheostomy

Tracheotomy, either percutaneous or surgical, may be performed to provide a more secure airway, facilitate a reduction in sedation, improve comfort and ultimately aid weaning from ventilation.

However, tracheostomy increases the risk of major haemorrhage, and this should be assessed in each patient. Early tracheostomy has not been shown to be associated with increased survival.

In selected patients, tracheal extubation (with or without non-invasive ventilation) can be considered, with the potential benefits of reducing the risks of oropharyngeal instrumentation and orotracheal intubation, improving communication and aiding compliance with rehabilitation.

Prone positioning

Prone positioning of adult patients on veno-venous ECMO may be considered. It can be done safely and effectively as long as great care is taken to secure all tubes and lines, and ensuring all pressure areas are well protected.

In addition to improving ventilation–perfusion relationships, it facilitates the drainage of pulmonary secretions, and may reduce right ventricular pressure overload and ventilator-associated lung injury.

Inhaled nitric oxide

Inhaled nitric oxide improves oxygenation in patients with acute lung injury by improving ventilation–perfusion matching and lowering pulmonary vascular resistance. Clinical trials have not demonstrated a mortality benefit, and it has no place in the management of the patient on veno-venous ECMO.

Key points

- Veno-venous ECMO allows gas exchange in the venous blood.
- The institution of least-damaging lung ventilation is thought to be beneficial.
- Patients can be extubated and breathe spontaneously on veno-venous ECMO.

TO LEARN MORE

Acute Respiratory Distress Syndrome Network (ARDSNet). (2000). Ventilation with lower tidal volumes as compared with traditional tidal volumes for acute lung injury and the acute respiratory distress syndrome. *New England Journal of Medicine*, 342, 1301–8.

Chapter 9

Management of the patient on veno-arterial ECMO: general principles

Introduction

Veno-arterial ECMO allows gas exchange and pumps blood from a vein to an artery. It is used to support failing lungs and can be used to support a failing heart.

Veno-arterial ECMO allows stabilization of the patient by perfusing vital organs with oxygenated blood. During veno-arterial ECMO, both the ECMO and the heart pump blood around the patient's body.

If no gas is flowing through the oxygenator, deoxygenated venous blood will be pumped into the arterial circulation, creating a veno-arterial shunt.

Veno-arterial ECMO will be continued until the clinical team has decided the best treatment for a specific patient. Two circulations having to work in parallel renders the management of the patient on veno-arterial ECMO much more complex than veno-venous ECMO. Patients may rapidly develop complications.

Patients supported with veno-arterial ECMO frequently have other organ failure and require a high level of critical care support. The day-to-day management of patients on veno-arterial ECMO is the same as for all critically ill patients, plus some specific elements. This chapter describes these specific elements.

Locally agreed protocols for the care of ECMO patients should be incorporated into training.

Monitoring of the patient on veno-arterial ECMO has been described in Chapter 4.

Stabilization on veno-arterial ECMO

Insertion of ECMO cannulas should ideally take place in an operating room. A variety of configurations can be used.

Peripheral cannulation can be achieved percutaneously and does not require surgery. Central and direct cannulation require surgery.

It can be striking how rapidly pharmacological support can be modified after veno-arterial ECMO support has been started. Inotropes and other vasoactive drugs can often be decreased.

It is essential to ensure that the heart continues to eject to avoid thrombosis in the cardiac cavities. Maintaining pulmonary blood flow may also prevent the formation of intrapulmonary thrombi. The absence of ventricular ejection will lead to cardiac distension and prevent possible cardiac recovery.

Lung ventilation can be adapted immediately after veno-arterial ECMO has been established. Similar principles of applying the least-damaging ventilation, as in veno-venous ECMO, should be applied (see Chapter 8). It is essential to ensure that the lungs still provide gas exchange, as the blood going through the lungs will need to be oxygenated (and CO_2 removed) to avoid a hypoxic mixture being delivered to some tissues (e.g. the coronary arteries). Changes in mechanical ventilation can affect the venous return and modify both cardiac output and ECMO flow.

After stabilization, the patient can undergo multiple non-invasive tests to determine the cause and decide subsequent management.

Oxygenation during veno-arterial ECMO

During veno-arterial ECMO support, O_2-saturated blood from the ECMO circuit enters the arterial circulation.

The PaO_2 in the arterial system at the point of entry is similar to that after the oxygenator, and it is therefore essential to adjust the O_2 concentration of the sweep gas going through the oxygenator.

The blood returning from the ECMO circuit will mix with any blood pumped by the heart. This will occur in the ascending aorta when central veno-arterial ECMO is used, or in any location if the ECMO blood is returned in a peripheral artery. There will be different concentrations of O_2 in different tissues. Arterial blood gases are ideally obtained from the right radial artery, as this will be the furthest accessible point of arterial blood when the ECMO blood is returned in the femoral artery.

Systemic arterial oxygenation is determined by the relative contributions of the native and ECMO circulation, ECMO blood flow, deoxygenated venous return, the degree of pulmonary dysfunction, O_2 consumption and oxygenator efficiency.

Adjuncts to veno-arterial ECMO

Leg reperfusion

In the case of peripheral ECMO, insertion of a reperfusion line is indispensable; this is described in Chapter 6.

Fluid balance

Removing excess water optimizes lung mechanics and pulmonary gas exchange but should be balanced against the need to keep the heart ejecting without excess distension.

Tracheostomy

Tracheostomy, either percutaneous or surgical, may be performed to provide a more secure airway, facilitate a reduction in sedation, improve comfort and ultimately aid weaning from ventilation.

However, tracheostomy increases the risk of major haemorrhage, and this should be assessed in each patient. Early tracheostomy has not been shown to be associated with increased survival.

It is often possible, and arguably preferable, to wake and extubate patients supported with veno-arterial ECMO.

Inotropes

Inotropes will be used to ensure the heart continues to eject. There is no evidence that continued use of inotropes facilitates recovery.

Intra-aortic balloon pump

An intra-aortic balloon pump may have been in place before the initiation of veno-arterial ECMO and continued afterwards. It may be inserted after initiation of veno-arterial ECMO to facilitate cardiac ejection.

Ventricular vents

The surgical insertion of ventricular vents might be required in the case of very poor remaining cardiac function with no ejection. This will prevent overdistension of the cardiac chambers and blood stasis with formation of thrombi. Blood will drain directly into the drainage side of the ECMO circuit. Extra cannulas increase the risk of disconnection or cannula displacement.

Another solution to a non-ejecting heart is to switch from peripheral veno-arterial ECMO to a central configuration. The direction of central veno-arterial ECMO blood flow does not increase the afterload and surgical vents can be inserted under direct vision.

Key points

- Management of the patient on veno-arterial ECMO is highly complex.
- Veno-arterial ECMO is only temporary and is used as a bridge to another solution or recovery.

TO LEARN MORE

Pellegrino V, Hockings LE, Davies A. (2014). Veno-arterial extracorporeal membrane oxygenation for adult cardiovascular failure. *Current Opinion in Critical Care*, 20, 484–92.

Soleimani B, Pae WE. (2012). Management of left ventricular distension during peripheral extracorporeal membrane oxygenation for cardiogenic shock. *Perfusion*, 27, 326–31.

Chapter 10

Patient transfer

The development of compact ECMO consoles and simpler circuits has made the transfer of patients supported with ECMO easier. However, there are still risks, including cannula dislodgement, console failure and bleeding.

The majority of patients requiring ECMO support will need to be transferred. This may only be to the operating room or the CT scan room within the hospital, or it may be from a referring centre to a unit able to provide ECMO support. It is possible for patients supported with ECMO to be moved from hospital to hospital, having been stabilized before transfer.

Some countries have set up networks based on a small number of high-volume centres working together to provide safe and efficient ECMO transfer. Clear guidelines and good communication between team members minimize the risk. All transfers require specific equipment, specially trained staff and planning to avoid potential mishap.

Planning

All transfers of patients on ECMO requires planning. Careful documentation is required and checklists are helpful.

Patients should be stabilized before transfer. This will require time. All lines should be secured. Non-essential medications should be interrupted. Replacement syringes must be prepared. Drugs and fluids that will need to be administered during transfer should be prepared and ready to be given when appropriate.

Emergency equipment should be checked before transfer. All batteries should be fully charged, and spares available when appropriate (power cables should accompany the patient).

Transfer team

Personnel included in the transfer of patients on ECMO vary from centre to centre. The team should be led by an intensive care doctor trained in the transfer of the critically ill patient. A person with intimate knowledge of the ECMO circuit, and trained in handling complications such as air embolism or circuit leakage, should accompany the patient at all times.

When retrieving patients not yet on ECMO, the doctor should have experience in cannulating and commencing ECMO support.

The team leader is responsible for the safety of team members and the patient during transfer. The team leader ensures communication between all team members to minimize the risk of complications.

Coordination at the ECMO centre is very important, ensuring that all runs smoothly. This includes being prepared for the team's return.

Transfer equipment

Transferring a patient on ECMO requires much specialized equipment. Patients are usually attached to a ventilator, multiple pieces of monitoring equipment with associated connections and multiple infusion pumps with associated indwelling vascular lines. All are critical to life and cannot be disconnected.

Patients can be transferred on a critical care bed, with modifications to accommodate the equipment described above plus the components of the ECMO circuit and required gas cylinders.

A transfer trolley can be modified to accommodate the ECMO consoles, oxygenator and circuit (Figure 10.1). Newer ECMO consoles often have specially designed transfer trolleys with fixation for the motor, console, oxygenator and O_2 cylinders. The extra weight needs to be taken into

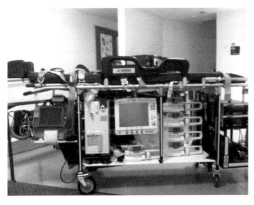

Figure 10.1 A transfer trolley modified to include ECMO consoles.

account, as this may limit the weight of the patient the trolley can support.

Appropriate mattresses are required in patients with a high risk of skin damage.

Replacement equipment is required in case of unexpected failure. This should include a back-up pump, driven either electrically or manually. A spare oxygenator and circuit are necessary.

Other resuscitation equipment such as suction systems and defibrillator are required.

Adequate power and an O_2 supply are required for the duration of the transfer. This means that vehicles or aircraft may need to be modified to accommodate the extra gas requirements, or be able to deliver the proper current. In vehicles, all equipment has to be secured to protect staff and patients.

When planning to cannulate and commence the ECMO in another hospital, the team needs to have enough equipment to accommodate the needs of the patient, including a variety of cannulas. All the equipment should be ready at all times, and checklists used to ensure nothing is missing.

Checklists should be available to support the team. This includes a World Health Organization insertion checklist to be used before inserting the cannula.

Care during transfer

Patient vital signs should be monitored during transfer. This includes heart rate and rhythm, blood pressure, O_2 saturation, end-tidal CO_2, temperature and pupil reaction.

The ECMO circuit must be monitored; this includes circuit pressure, sweep gas and pump flow monitoring. All observations should be regularly documented. Portable devices allow monitoring of blood gases and coagulation during long transfers.

Transfer by air

The advantage of air transfer is reduced journey time. This is essential in some countries. Transfer by air is more expensive than by road, with helicopter usually being the most expensive form of transfer. Staff require special training.

The logistical and organizational requirements often mean that it is impractical if the planned journey is less than 2 h, as transferring between several vehicles is often required. Very few hospitals have an airstrip in their grounds, but many have a helipad close by.

Space is often limited, as well as the mode of entry to the cabin. Patients on ECMO may not fit through the door or in the cabin of an aircraft. Pressure bags should be available as the space in the cabin does not usually allow infusion by gravity. Acceleration, deceleration and frequent bumps during flight can all disturb the patient, equipment and infusions.

With altitude, gas will expand. This may affect a pneumothorax and other bubbles in the patient or the ECMO circuit. The endotracheal tube cuff should be filled with saline to avoid hyperinflation and tracheal damage. The balloon of a pulmonary artery catheter should be emptied. The altitude will affect the gas-exchange capacity of the membrane.

If using a helicopter, the noise level is very high. Auscultation is not possible. Audible monitoring appears silent. Conversation is impossible without aid. All patients should have earplugs.

The safety of the team is paramount, and flying should never be attempted if the pilot thinks it is inappropriate.

Key points

- Transferring the patient on ECMO aims to ensure continuity of intensive care support during the whole journey.
- Transferring on ECMO has risks and requires planning and communication.
- Air transport is possible, but space is often limited and limiting.

TO LEARN MORE

Biscotti M, Agerstrand C, Abrams D, *et al.* (2015). One hundred transports on extracorporeal support to an extracorporeal membrane oxygenation center. *Annals of Thoracic Surgery*, 100, 34–9.

Intensive Care Society. (2011). *Guidelines for the Transport of the Critically Ill Adult*, 3rd edn. London: Intensive Care Society.

Chapter 11

Liberation from ECMO

Introduction

No one can remain on ECMO for ever. The goal should be to remove ECMO at the earliest opportunity.

In veno-venous ECMO, lung recovery will be awaited and liberation from ECMO support sought on a daily basis. It is striking how poor clinicians can be at predicting residual physiological reserves in patients. Veno-venous ECMO is particularly well suited to demonstrate this again and again at the bedside. A small number of patients may never be liberated and may be bridged to a lung transplant.

Veno-arterial ECMO is a support that gives time to the clinical team to evaluate the best next options. It can sometimes be used to bridge a patient to recovery but will usually allow stabilization and evaluation in preparation for other forms of treatment or support.

Liberating the patient on veno-venous ECMO

An easy test to assess patient readiness is to disconnect the gas sweep from the oxygenator (note: this should *never* be done in veno-arterial ECMO). All gas exchange will then have to be done by the patient's lungs. Blood will simply circulate through the ECMO circuit with no consequence other than the mechanical stress imposed on its components. Veno-venous ECMO without a gas sweep can be continued for hours without any impact on a recovered patient. It can also be reinitiated at the 'flick of a switch' by starting the gas sweep.

Some centres will incorporate a daily automatic test off sweep. It is often surprising to see patients being able to ventilate fully despite being deemed too sick by the clinical team.

Clinical improvement is suggested by an improvement in lung compliance (estimated from tidal volume and pressure measured on the ventilator), radiological appearances, gas exchange and laboratory parameters.

Some clinicians advocate that there is no such action as weaning from the ECMO circuit, while others will advocate that a progressive wean can be instituted. This is similar to the discussions surrounding weaning a patient from a ventilator, and experience will differ from centre to centre.

Clinical adjustment to flow and sweep are continuously required to meet physiological targets while the patient is treated. ECMO flow will be decreased when the patient's own oxygenation is improving (improved lung function or lower cardiac output). The gas sweep is affected by so many factors that it is wrong to believe it is a marker of progress in patient status. An example of a chart used to manage the pump and use the lowest possible setting is shown in Figure 11.1.

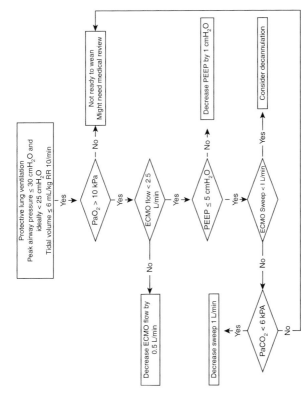

Figure 11.1 A veno-venous ECMO weaning algorithm. Example of an algorithm used by staff at the bedside to decrease the level of ventilatory support in patients on veno-venous ECMO. RR, respiratory rate.

If the patient has been supported adequately and lung function has recovered sufficiently, the ECMO can be removed.

Liberating the patient on veno-arterial ECMO

Liberating a patient from veno-arterial ECMO is usually a complex exercise, except when it simply entails moving to another form of mechanical support.

If the heart has fully recovered, it will be obvious that the two circulations are competing. The patient can then be taken to the operating room for the arterial cannula to be removed under direct surgical vision (blind removal of a percutaneous cannula is possible but not as safe).

If it is unsure that the heart recovery is sufficient to sustain physiological demand, there is no universal protocol. Similar measures to those used to come off cardiopulmonary bypass are used, and an expert team is required.

One key difference compared with cardiopulmonary bypass is that in veno-arterial ECMO the liberation attempt can be stopped while the team review plans, including the possibility of non-reversibility or long-term support.

Various protocols have been proposed and several indices suggested as indicators of success, but none replaces experienced cardiac surgical teams in this endeavour.

End-of-life care

Mortality in patients receiving ECMO remains high, and clinicians will often have to manage the end of a life.

This can be extremely difficult in situations where the pump is keeping the patient alive and there is no possibility of progression to further treatment or support. Patients may be fully awake and aware, and support to them, their family and the staff is necessary.

Clear and consistent communication between the ECMO team and families, balancing hopes of recovery with realistic estimates of the risk of dying, is key in preparing for difficult decisions at the end of life. Involvement of specialist palliative care physicians and nurses can be very valuable.

Many patients may have recorded a prior wish to consider organ donation, and the opportunity to discuss potential organ and/or tissue donation should be offered. This is done in accordance with local guidance.

Key points

- Liberation from veno-venous ECMO can follow protocol.
- Interruption of the gas sweep in patients on veno-venous ECMO is a good test to assess whether ECMO is still required.
- Gas sweep should *never* be interrupted in patients on veno-arterial ECMO.
- Liberation from veno-arterial ECMO is easy when obvious, but complex and unsure when not.

TO LEARN MORE

Cui WW, Ramsey JG. (2015). Pharmacologic approaches to weaning from cardiopulmonary bypass and extracorporeal membrane oxygenation. *Best Practice and Research Clinical Anaesthesiology*, 29, 257–70.

Licker M, Diaper J, Cartier V, *et al.* (2012). Clinical review: management of weaning from cardiopulmonary bypass after cardiac surgery. *Annals of Cardiac Anaesthesia*, 15, 206–23.

Chapter 12

Specifics of intensive care management for the patient on ECMO

All principles of intensive care management apply to the patient on ECMO. Some aspects need special consideration. These are discussed in this chapter.

Sedation and paralysis

Most patients are heavily sedated and often paralysed when ECMO support is started.

Muscle relaxants should be discontinued at the earliest opportunity. The risk of awareness is increased in patients with a sudden change in the volume of distribution of drugs when ECMO is commenced.

Continued sedation is not required to support a patient with ECMO and should be discontinued at the earliest opportunity. Most patients will, however, require sedation for several days, often in the context of distressing multiorgan failure and an intense inflammatory response.

The pharmacokinetics and bioavailability of most drugs seem to be modified, but little is known about the specifics (see Pharmacology and ECMO, this chapter).

Analgesia must be continued and titrated to provide comfort and allow pain-free interventions and nursing care.

The presence of ECMO renders daily sedation breaks easier, as the respiratory drive can be controlled by adjusting CO_2 removal. Interrupting the sedation allows an assessment of neurological function. This is a key step in ensuring that ECMO is not futile, for example in patients with neurological injuries such as an intracranial bleed.

Ventilation and haemodynamic support during ECMO

These are discussed extensively in most other chapters of this book.

Renal function and ECMO

Acute kidney injury (AKI) is common in patients supported with ECMO, with approximately 50% requiring renal replacement therapy (RRT).

The need for RRT may reflect inadequate renal perfusion or may result from a direct injury to the kidneys. These can be caused by the underlying insult, such as sepsis, respiratory failure or cardiac failure with high vasopressor requirements. If the insult is short lived, the kidneys can recover fully. Renal replacement therapy can be used to manage fluid balance in these very ill patients.

The criteria for starting RRT used for other critically ill patients are applicable to the patient supported with ECMO. These include significant acidaemia (pH <7.25), hyperkalaemia resistant to other therapy, pulmonary oedema due to fluid overload, and significant uraemia. There is no consensus regarding the optimal timing of RRT in patients with AKI, and this extends to the patient supported with ECMO.

The management of RRT is similar to that used in all critically ill patients.

Impact of ECMO on renal function

The rapid haemodynamic changes altering renal blood flow may cause ischaemia or trigger a reperfusion injury in the kidney. This can lead to AKI.

Table 12.1 lists the possible causes of AKI during ECMO.

A high arterial blood pressure not responding to treatment is often observed in ECMO patients. The mechanism is unknown but is possibly multifactorial. Contributing factors include fluid retention, a reduction in nitric oxide plasma level (due to an increase in the level of plasma-free haemoglobin mediating nitric oxide scavenging), variation in blood levels of drugs and a possible alteration of the renin–angiotensin system.

Table 12.1 Possible causes of AKI during ECMO

Non-pulsatile arterial blood flow (in veno-arterial ECMO)
Inflammatory response
Hypercoaguable state
Haemolysis
Possible high level of blood product transfusion

Indications for RRT in patients treated with ECMO

The combination of ECMO and RRT has several potential benefits: it allows optimization of the fluid balance, which permits the administration of adequate nutrition, intravenous drugs and blood products by preventing fluid overload; and it may decrease the inflammatory response.

Most ECMO patients will receive RRT either because of worsening renal failure (as indicated by the biochemistry results) or to control their fluid balance. Timely administration of fluids is life-saving, but fluid in excess will have a negative effect on outcome.

Patients will often not tolerate significant fluid removal immediately after initiation of ECMO, probably due to the intense capillary leak resulting from the inflammatory response. Eventually it will be possible to filter out large volumes, and this will be beneficial in relation to cardiac and/or lung recovery.

ECMO blood flow may be compromised by RRT if the filtration rate is excessive. An intravascular volume depletion can be observed in patients on RRT, and this may precipitate pre-renal azotemia, subsequent AKI and lengthening of the duration of ECMO support. We usually advocate removing a maximum of 2 L of fluid over 24 h in an average 70 kg person and aim to return to the pre-disease weight.

The patient's condition will ultimately affect how fluid management is conducted and how the patient may respond to fluid shifts.

Methods of RRT during ECMO support

Renal replacement therapy can be conducted with continuous peritoneal dialysis. This provides less effective clearance of electrolyte and waste products. Intra-abdominal haemorrhage can be an issue.

Intravascular access for RRT can be provided via a separate dedicated central venous catheter. This allows RRT to be continued once ECMO support is removed.

Introduction of a haemofiltration filter into the ECMO circuit is possible. The filter inlet is connected after the pump, and the blood can be returned at various points in the circuit. This system provides slow continuous ultrafiltration, and continuous convective clearance with replacement fluids is possible. The technique is simple, cheap and uses a smaller blood volume than a conventional machine. It carries a significant risk of monitoring error with uncontrolled volume shifts or sudden failure of the haemofilter. Access by connecting to the ECMO circuit is possible (Figure 12.1). This is necessary where vascular access is difficult. It is the preferred method in some centres. One option is to connect the RRT device to the inlet and outlet ports of the oxygenator. The inflow of RRT is connected to the arterial tubing of the ECMO circuit just after the oxygenator and the outflow to the tubing of the ECMO circuit just before the oxygenator. The system returns the blood to the oxygenator.

The RRT circuit may need to be reconfigured slightly to take account of access and return vascular pressures, as the

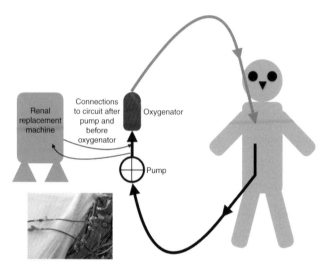

Figure 12.1 Connection of the RRT machine to the ECMO circuit.

machine safety mechanisms may not allow the use of high-pressure systems. Connection and disconnection from the ECMO circuit increases the risk of air entrainment, leakage and infection. It is important to remember that air can be entrained in the ECMO circuit from any indwelling vascular line open to the air. Connection of the RRT device to the ECMO venous circuit (Figure 12.1) allows the use of all the potential modes including continuous veno-venous haemofiltration, continuous veno-venous haemodialysis and continuous veno-venous haemodiafiltration.

Connecting the return blood from the continuous RRT device to the tubing before the oxygenator allows air and thrombi to be trapped in the oxygenator, and avoids venous admixture into the oxygenated tubing of the ECMO circuit. Connecting a full RRT system allows accurate monitoring of any mode of filtration, increases the accuracy of fluid balance and keeps a constant blood flow through the filter. Finally, filters can easily be changed without disruption of the ECMO flow.

Renal replacement therapy can be performed by connecting the RRT device to the venous line before the centrifugal pump, but this low negative pressure increases the risk of haemolysis and microembolization. Air embolism is more likely to happen at the time of connection/disconnection.

Independent vascular access can be used. The advantages of this approach include less interference with the ECMO circuit. The insertion of a large catheter in an anticoagulated patient increases the risk of bleeding. Veins may already be in use with other lines. It is important that impaired cerebral venous return is considered in patients with large catheters inserted in all neck vessels. The RRT circuit and vascular catheters can be a source of major air embolism, even when not directly connected to the ECMO circuit.

Anticoagulation with RRT and ECMO

The anticoagulation used in patients with ECMO is sufficient to prevent thrombi forming in the RRT circuit. Additional anticoagulation is not routinely used.

If ECMO support is provided without systemic anticoagulation, the RRT circuit is at high risk of occlusion with thrombi (the blood flow through an RRT circuit is much lower than in the ECMO circuit). Techniques reliant on the anticoagulant running exclusively in the RRT circuits are possible (such as citrate anticoagulation).

Plasmapheresis

Plasmapheresis can easily be conducted during ECMO by using a compatible RRT machine and connecting it to the ECMO circuit as described above.

Sepsis on ECMO

ECMO during refractory septic shock

Septic shock in the adult patient is usually associated with low systemic vascular resistance and refractory hypotension with preserved cardiac output. This distributive shock is related to a maldistribution of blood flow at a microvascular level, and veno-arterial ECMO is of little value in restoring vascular tone.

This is different from what is observed in children, and the international guidelines for the management of severe sepsis and septic shock in children recommends considering veno-arterial ECMO for circulatory collapse unresponsive to all conventional treatment. This remains controversial in adult patients suffering from refractory septic shock. Veno-arterial ECMO might prove useful if the cause of the shock is cardiogenic in addition to distributive.

Nosocomial infections in patients supported with ECMO

There is a long definition of nosocomial infection in patients supported with ECMO: an infection not present at the start of support but detected more than 24 h after ECMO commencement, or within the first 48 h after ECMO discontinuation, and with a pathogen different from those detected within 7 days before ECMO initiation.

The risk of infection is markedly increased in the patient supported with ECMO because of the presence of multiple indwelling devices. Activation of the inflammatory response by the ECMO circuit, coupled with the primary insult, often leads to a relatively immunosuppressed status that may decrease the ability to respond to secondary insults.

Nosocomial infection is the second most common complication of ECMO after haemorrhage, and affects up to two-thirds of patients supported by ECMO. Ventilator-associated pneumonia and bloodstream infections are the most common causes, followed by surgical wounds, urinary tract infection and cannulation-related infection.

The most commonly identified organisms include coagulase-negative *Staphylococcus, Pseudomonas aeruginosa, Staphylococcus aureus* and *Candida albicans. Enterobacter, Klebsiella, Enterococcus* and *Escherichia coli* species are also possible.

The risk of nosocomial infection is increased if the ECMO support is continued for a long time, in cases of mechanical complication, if the patient has an autoimmune disease and if veno-venous ECMO is used.

All the standard measures used in intensive care to decrease the risk of nosocomial infections are applicable. Elevation of the head of the bed, oral prophylaxis and medical treatment of reflux should be strictly followed. All unnecessary lines should be removed. Strict aseptic techniques should be used to access all indwelling catheters.

The diagnosis of newly acquired infection can be challenging because of the intense inflammatory response that mimics sepsis itself. The temperature of the blood is maintained by the circuit's heat exchanger, and fever can easily be masked. Physical examination and radiographic changes may be difficult to interpret. Subtle changes in clinical condition and signs of poor perfusion manifested by metabolic acidosis, increasing lactate levels, decreasing urine output and a rise in hepatic transaminases are all indices of possible sepsis.

Blood, urine and tracheal cultures should be obtained from patients on ECMO at the earliest suspicion of a possible secondary infection.

Antibiotic therapy

The principles of good antibiotic stewardship apply to all critically ill patients, and include appropriate initial therapy, regular reviews, de-escalation where possible, appropriate prophylaxis, and use of local guidelines and specialist advice.

Treatment of documented infections should follow the same principles as for patients who are not on ECMO support. The increased volume of distribution and impaired drug clearance may affect the dosage of antibiotics. Drug level monitoring in the blood is appropriate where possible.

The underlying diagnosis in the majority of patients who receive ECMO for severe acute respiratory failure is bacterial or viral pneumonia, although a definitive microbiological diagnosis is not reached in approximately one-third of patients. Antibiotic therapy for severe pneumonia should initially be broad spectrum and then more focused when a definitive microbiological diagnosis is reached. National and local patterns of disease and antimicrobial resistance will guide initial and subsequent therapy, and local advice should be sought.

It is common practice to administer single-dose prophylactic antibiotics on ECMO cannulation, decannulation and when changing components of the ECMO circuit, although there is limited evidence to support this.

Pharmacology and ECMO

Effective treatment of the primary disease and subsequent complications is required in order to cure those patients supported with ECMO.

Drug pharmacokinetics may be altered in patients on ECMO because of an increased volume of distribution and reduced drug clearance, due at least in part to the binding of drugs to the ECMO circuit (Figure 12.2).

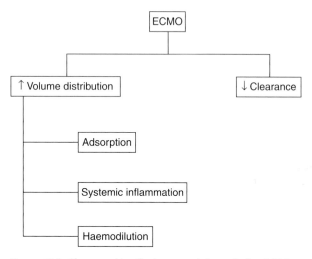

Figure 12.2 Pharmacokinetic changes of drugs during ECMO.

It is not possible to predict the effect of ECMO on pharmacokinetics, and it is impossible to integrate this with the effects of critical illness, drug interactions and RRT.

Therapeutic drug monitoring helps prevent toxicity and monitor efficacy.

Intravenous drugs should be administered directly to the patient and not via the ECMO circuit. This reduces the risks of air entrainment during manipulation of the connectors, or inadvertent rapid drug delivery due to negative pressure in the drainage limb of the circuit. Clotting factors and lipid-rich solutions, such as propofol and parenteral nutrition, should not be given directly in the ECMO circuit, as the high concentration of lipids may block the oxygenator.

Drug availability changes during ECMO

The ECMO circuit will increase the volume of distribution because its material can bind circulating proteins and drugs. This will be affected by the type of components used in the circuit. Reduced adsorption is observed in hollow-fibre oxygenator membranes. Less adsorption is observed in circuits with shorter tubing and those using centrifugal pumps. Drug molecular size, degree of ionization, lipophilicity and plasma protein binding may also influence the adsorption to circuit components.

Adsorption of lipophilic drugs to ECMO membranes and tubing is common and likely to rapidly reduce plasma concentrations. Highly lipophilic drugs such as fentanyl or midazolam will disappear almost completely in an ECMO circuit. However, not all drugs are affected, and the extent of sequestration is not consistent.

The volume of the ECMO circuit increases the total blood volume, and this is compounded by the haemodilution due to repeated blood transfusions, loss in the circulating blood volume during changes in the equipment and the administration of fluids to maintain ECMO flow. This will mainly affect hydrophilic drugs.

The inflammatory response induced by the exposure of blood to foreign material and sepsis causes a redistribution of albumin that is disproportionate, resulting in a low plasma albumin concentration. The proportion of unbound drugs is then increased, with a higher extravascular distribution.

Prolonged elimination is multifactorial, but the reduction of renal function is the primary determinant. Prolonged half-lives of gentamicin and vancomycin are seen in ECMO patients, and meropenem will often remain at a higher level. Adding haemofiltration or other modes of continuous RRT to the ECMO device may increase drug clearance, but this is disputed.

Regional blood flow changes in the liver during pulseless veno-arterial ECMO can also affect clearance of those drugs with a high extraction ratio, such as propranolol.

A decreased drug elimination rate predisposes patients to toxicity, especially for the drugs with a narrow therapeutic window.

Available pharmacokinetic studies have many limitations because they have been performed ex vivo and in neonates with immature enzymatic and elimination systems.

A summary of the changes in pharmacokinetic caused by the ECMO circuit is shown in Table 12.2.

A few specific drugs and ECMO

Many of the statements in this section are assumptions based on in vitro studies or observations in the paediatric population. They are important enough to appear in a book about ECMO in the adult patient. They also illustrate the great variability and unknowns when using them in a patient on ECMO support.

Ex vivo studies have demonstrated significant loss of **fentanyl, diazepam, lorazepam** and **midazolam** in an

Table 12.2 Pharmacokinetic changes during ECMO support

Factor	Change	Therapeutic outcome	Drugs
Haemodilution (priming of the circuit, blood transfusions)	↑ Vd	↑ Loading dose, dosage frequency	Hydrophilic drugs, highly protein-bound drugs
Adsorbtion in the ECMO circuit	↑ Vd	↑ Loading dose,	Lipophilic drugs
Systemic inflammation or/and sepsis	↑ Vd	↑ Loading dose	Hydrophilic drugs
Organ failures	↓ CL	↓ Dosage frequency	Renal or liver elimination

Vd, volume of distribution; Cl, clearance.

ECMO circuit. **Morphine** is less absorbed and therefore preferred.

Acetaminophen (**paracetamol**) is significantly less lipophilic and protein bound than **fentanyl**.

Propofol is a widely used, short-acting, hypnotic agent and is significantly sequestrated in the ECMO circuit.

Dexmedetomidine is a highly lipophilic α2-receptor agonist and up to 90% of the drug is lost in an ECMO circuit.

Vancomycin and **gentamicin** have an increased volume of distribution. Elimination half-lives for both drugs are prolonged during ECMO, and several studies have demonstrated a return to expected values after cessation of ECMO. Ex vivo studies did not find significant loss of vancomycin in the ECMO circuit.

No significant differences between ECMO and non-ECMO patients in serum concentrations, volume of distribution, total clearance and half-life has been found for **meropenem** and **piperacillin**.

Most drugs that are not usually highly protein bound or do not show a high degree of lipophilicity remain relatively stable in the ECMO circuit.

Caspofungin is freely water soluble and therefore sequestration to the ECMO circuit is not expected. Plasma caspofungin levels using loading and daily maintenance doses of 70 mg do not differ between ECMO and non-ECMO patients.

Voriconazole, a highly lipophilic drug, is significantly sequestered in the circuit, necessitating initial higher doses of the drug, which must later be reduced due to possible circuit saturation to avoid drug toxicity.

Suboptimal plasma concentrations of **neuraminidase inhibitors** may be associated with reduced antiviral effectiveness of the drug and the development of viral drug resistance. However, the pharmacokinetics of **oseltamivir** does not seem to be significantly influenced during ECMO support.

The estimated clearance for **theophylline** is significantly lower and the volume of distribution higher; these differences are probably a result of the expanded circulating volume during ECMO and altered renal and hepatic physiology. The increased volume of distribution and long half-life suggest that an initial loading dose is necessary, with the reduction of the maintenance dose to avoid toxic concentrations.

Furosemide is lost in the circuit components, but there seems to be no difference between intermittent and continuous administration.

Ranitidine is not affected.

Anti-epileptic drugs such as **phenobarbital** and **phenytoin** are highly sequestrated in the ECMO circuit. A higher phenobarbital loading and maintenance dose may be required during ECMO support. **Levetiracetam** is a first-line therapy for seizures in critically ill patients because of its clinical efficacy, minimal drug interactions and wide therapeutic window. It is hydrophilic and has minimal protein binding, and indeed does not seem to be affected by ECMO.

Amiodarone is highly lipophilic and is likely to be sequestered in the ECMO circuit. Higher doses may be needed. No changes are required in dosing **hydralazine. Nicardipine** requires higher doses due to the larger volume of distribution.

More than one-half of administered **heparin** is eliminated by the extracorporeal circuit itself or by blood components in the circuit.

Cyclosporine and **insulin** are likely to bind to the ECMO circuit.

Nutrition during ECMO

Malnutrition is associated with increased morbidity and mortality in critically ill patients. This is no different for the patient supported with ECMO.

Patients on ECMO demonstrate a marked catabolic stress response.

Patients on ECMO present several risk factors for peptic ulceration including multiple organ failure, coagulopathy, administration of corticosteroids and difficulties in establishing enteral feeding. Ulcer prophylaxis with a histamine type 2 receptor blocker or proton pump inhibitor is indicated.

Significant nasopharyngeal bleeding can be caused by the insertion of nasogastric tubes in patients supported with ECMO. The orogastric route may be a preferred option.

Metabolism and energy requirements for patients on ECMO

The metabolic response to illness is associated with a persistent increase of insulin concentration, catecholamine, glucagon and cortisol. Increased levels of cytokines released by activated macrophages promote catabolism and are associated with increased mortality.

Patients requiring support with ECMO usually present with an accentuated breakdown of skeletal muscle protein (the hallmark of the catabolic response to critical illness). This protein breakdown is required to provide gluconeogenesis, amino acids for the synthesis of acute-phase proteins and proteins for tissue repair. The progressive loss of skeletal muscle protein leads to respiratory compromise, cardiac dysfunction and increased susceptibility to infection.

Once the patient is liberated from ECMO, the caloric requirement needs adjusting. This is best achieved by measuring the energy expenditure using an indirect calorimeter, although this is rarely done in practice.

Nutrition initiation time and mode of delivery for ECMO patients

Adequate nutritional support in ECMO patients is challenging because of an active ongoing metabolic stress response, the clinical requirements for fluid restriction and often an intolerance of enteral feeding.

Early establishment of enteral nutrition is desirable in patients supported with ECMO. Enteral nutrition improves nitrogen balance, prevents gut mucosal atrophy, decreases frequency of bacterial translocation, improves immune function and reduces overall cost. Gastric feeding via a nasogastric tube is the preferred route. Jejunal tube placement should be considered if feed is not absorbed.

Various observational studies confirm that enteral nutrition at approximately 25 kcal/kg/day can be achieved within a week of initiation of either veno-venous and veno-arterial ECMO. This can be done in prone patients.

Controversies exist regarding the route of administration and time of initiation in haemodynamically unstable patients.

The two main barriers for delivery of enteral nutrition are interruption for a procedure and a high gastric residual volume. This can be solved by implementing strict protocols including the use of prokinetics allowing higher gastric residual volume, using post-pyloric feeding tubes and nursing the patient with their head elevated at 45°. Interruption of feed for procedures should be considered carefully. These interruptions can be decreased substantially with adequate planning and reassurance that some procedures will not need fasting as the stomach contents can be aspirated.

If tolerance of enteral feed decreases below 50% for at least 24 h after 1 week of ECMO, parenteral nutrition should be initiated but stopped as soon as absorption of enteral feed is greater than 75%.

Parenteral nutrition may be required in patients who cannot tolerate enteral nutrition. There is a theoretical risk of damage to the oxygenator from lipid-rich parenteral nutrition products, but this is very rarely seen in practice.

The volume of feed adds substantially to the overall amount of fluid administered to patients. This should be carefully considered and a compromise between volume and calories must sometimes be found.

Awake patients should be allowed to eat, but nutritional supplements might not be required.

Protein, carbohydrate and lipid requirements for ECMO patients

Critically ill patients supported with ECMO have a high protein turnover used to synthesize the proteins needed for the inflammatory response and tissue repair. Protein catabolism leads to a progressive loss of diaphragmatic, intercostal and cardiac muscle. Amino acid nutritional supplementation may reduce this overall negative protein balance. Patients receiving RRT have an even higher protein requirement due to amino acids lost through the filter.

Excessive protein administration should be avoided, especially in patients with marginal renal or liver function. Of note, enteral or parenteral glutamine supplementation in order to reduce the septic complications in critically ill patients is no longer recommended.

The catabolism of skeletal muscle generates glucose, as it is the preferred substrate for the brain, red blood cells and renal medulla, and provides the energy required by injured tissue. Septic patients have a threefold increase in glucose turnover, glucose oxidation and elevation of gluconeogenesis. Provision of dietary glucose is relatively ineffective in reducing gluconeogenesis. The excess glucose is converted to fat, resulting in the generation of CO_2. The normal ketone metabolism is impaired in the stressed metabolic state, thus making glucose the main fuel for the brain.

Lipid metabolism is accelerated in critically ill patients. The process involves the recycling of free fatty acid and glycerol into triglycerides. Approximately one-third of released fatty acids are oxidized to release energy, and this is the prime source of energy in stressed patients. The glycerol portion of the triglycerides may be converted to pyruvate and then metabolized to glucose. Provision of dietary glucose does not diminish lipid recycling.

Electrolyte plasma levels (potassium, sodium, calcium, chloride and bicarbonates) must be measured frequently. Fluid shifts, the catabolic response to illness and multiple drugs will cause changes in electrolyte levels.

Potassium shifts may cause arrhythmias. Hypophosphataemia may cause thrombocytopenia and respiratory muscle dysfunction. Hypomagnesaemia may be the cause of cardiac arrhythmias. Hypochloraemia can result in metabolic alkalosis that inhibits the respiratory drive, leading to a potassium intracellular shift and a decrease in circulating ionized calcium. Chloride can be administered through a parenteral nutrition formula.

The need for vitamins and trace elements in the ECMO patient is similar to that in the healthy population. Excessive dosage is a risk.

Renal replacement therapy is often used during ECMO (see Renal function and ECMO, this chapter). This will result in further replacement requirements, as in other critically ill patients supported with RRT.

Enteral nutrition-related complications

Adverse events related to enteral nutrition include pulmonary aspiration, nosocomial pneumonia and abdominal complications.

Decreased blood flow to the abdominal organs is associated with ischaemic injury, bacterial translocation and multiple organ failure. This may be exacerbated by vasoactive drugs administered in the context of the primary insult.

Signs of intolerance (abdominal distention, increasing nasogastric tube aspirate or gastric residual volumes, decreased passage of stool and flatus, hypoactive bowel sounds, increasing metabolic acidosis and/or base deficit) should be closely monitored.

Aperients should be used from initiation of ECMO.

Nursing on ECMO

Nursing of the patient on ECMO is similar to nursing of the complex critically ill patient.

Aside from the various points raised throughout this book, special attention should be given to positioning and the increased risk of pressure sores from cannulas and tubing (Figure 12.3).

Nurses will have a key role in the rehabilitation process (see Rehabilitation, this chapter).

Pressure from cannula side arm behind ear

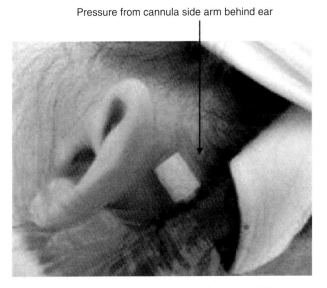

Figure 12.3 Risk of pressure sores is greatly increased in patients supported by ECMO.

Physiotherapy on ECMO

Patients on ECMO will require physiotherapy treatment as required. Physiotherapists will be part of the multidisciplinary team instituting rehabilitation (see Rehabilitation, this chapter), and ECMO patients should be assessed by a suitably qualified physiotherapist within a timely fashion.

Chest physiotherapy may be beneficial. It can reduce ventilator-associated pneumonia, improve static lung compliance, enhance sputum clearance, and address atelectasis and lobar collapse. The aim of chest physiotherapy is clearance of airway secretions in the early stages of admission and recruitment of lung volume in the later stages.

The only limitations to the treatment options that can be proposed are related to the ECMO circuit and anticoagulation.

Suction of the airways can cause life-threatening haemorrhage. Modification of intrathoracic pressure can affect ECMO blood flow. Cannula positioning may prevent adequate positioning.

Rehabilitation

There is increasing evidence showing that early rehabilitation of the critically ill patient leads to improved functional ability, decreased duration of mechanical ventilation, and decreased intensive care and duration of hospital stay. One could easily extrapolate that rehabilitation may decrease the duration of

ECMO support. Early intervention decreases the incidence of delirium and mortality.

ECMO patients often have had prolonged bed rest, increased use of muscle relaxants and increased use of steroids (sometimes initiated before ECMO has been considered). These factors increase the risk of physical disability secondary to immobility and critical illness.

A multidisciplinary approach to provide rehabilitation to complex patients is required, including staff with experience of mobilizing patients on ECMO. Patients can be rehabilitated with internal jugular or femoral cannulation. Venous cannulation usually allows out-of-bed mobilization. Arterial cannulation of the femoral arteries, with the presence of a femoral line, usually precludes mobilization out of bed. This is another reason to move on from peripheral ECMO at an early stage.

The location of the ECMO cannula may impede the extent of the rehabilitation. Security of the cannula should be paramount and the position continuously checked. An ECMO cannula should be adequately supported by the use of a headband, tapes or other fixations.

Mobilization will always require several members of the team, including nurses, a physiotherapist and specialists who understand the ECMO circuit and are able to deal with emergencies.

The rehabilitation process should be clearly explained to the patient and/or family, and the risks and benefits of rehabilitation made clear.

Involvement of occupational therapists, speech and language therapists, and psychologists should be considered early.

Key points

- ECMO support can be provided without sedation.
- The principles of RRT are the same with or without ECMO.
- The RRT circuit safely can be connected to the ECMO circuit.
- Drug monitoring is required and would be ideal for all drugs given to the patient on ECMO.
- Patients on ECMO demonstrate a marked catabolic stress response.

TO LEARN MORE

Askenazi DJ, Selewski DT, Paden ML, *et al.* (2012). Renal replacement therapy in critically ill patients receiving extracorporeal membrane oxygenation. *Clinical Journal of the American Society of Nephrology*, 7, 1328–36.

Jamal JA, Economou CJ, Lipman J, Roberts JA. (2012). Improving antibiotic dosing in special situations in the ICU: burns, renal replacement therapy and extracorporeal membrane oxygenation. *Current Opinion in Critical Care* 18, 460–71.

Wildschut ED, Ahsman MJ, Allegaert K, Mathot RA, Tibboel D. (2010). Determinants of drug absorption in different ECMO circuits. *Intensive Care Medicine*, 36, 2109–16.

Chapter 13

Extracorporeal carbon dioxide removal or ECCO$_2$R

Principles

Extracorporeal CO$_2$ removal (ECCO$_2$R) provides support for patients with severe acute respiratory failure characterized by hypercapnia with subsequent respiratory acidosis. It can be used to support a low mechanical ventilation strategy by supporting CO$_2$ clearance.

An ECCO$_2$R circuit consists of tubing allowing the blood to flow through a plastic module containing a diffusion membrane (comprising built-in multiple hollow fibres to increase the surface area). The circuit is usually heparin coated to reduce thrombus formation and is resistant to plasma leakage. The blood flows on one side of the membrane and the sweep gas on the other. Increasing the rate of the sweep gas will increase the amount of CO$_2$ eliminated.

The principle of ECCO$_2$R is based on the fact that lower blood flows are required to exchange CO$_2$ across a diffusion membrane (while maintaining sweep gas flow). The quantity of CO$_2$ that can be exchanged is at least as high as that produced by the metabolism.

Using lower blood flows allows the use of smaller cannulas and decreases the overall risk.

During ECCO$_2$R, O$_2$ will be exchanged if O$_2$ is added in the sweep gas. Oxygen will diffuse across the membrane, with the blood exiting the ECCO$_2$R circuit being oxygenated. This will usually be insignificant to the patient, as this oxygenated blood will immediately be diluted with a higher volume of deoxygenated blood. If oxygenation is sought, higher blood flows are required and this is then ECMO.

Clearing CO$_2$ reduces the ventilation required and therefore decreases ventilator-induced lung injury in the mechanically ventilated patient. The use of ECCO$_2$R can prevent intubation or support liberation from a ventilator.

Using ECCO$_2$R can be a bridge to lung transplantation and can support patients presenting with acute or chronic lung conditions (e.g. pneumonia in the patient with chronic obstructive pulmonary disease).

The low flow used during ECCO$_2$R requires continuous anticoagulation. It is noteworthy that thrombi will develop more rapidly in these systems than in ECMO, due to the lower blood flow.

Devices used for ECCO$_2$R

Arterio-venous ECCO$_2$R

Arterio-venous ECCO$_2$R utilizes the patient's arterio-venous pressure gradient to pump blood through the membrane. Access is most commonly achieved with a percutaneous cannulation of the femoral artery and vein.

These systems are reliant on the patient's blood pressure to pump the blood through the circuit, and a mean arterial blood pressure of greater than 60 mmHg is required to achieve flow rates between 0.5 and 1.2 L/min.

The resistance to blood flow is low, but build-up from a thrombus in the membrane may progressively increase the resistance to flow, and higher pressures will be required to maintain an adequate flow.

The advantages of this system include the ease of cannula insertion, which can be done in the ICU using ultrasound guidance. In addition, due to the simplicity of the design allowing the membrane lung to be positioned on the bed between the patient's legs, it is easily transportable.

The inability to mobilize the patient due to femoral arterial cannulation is one disadvantage of using arterio-venous ECCO$_2$R.

The main risk is distal limb ischaemia, which can occur on the side of the arterial cannulation. The possible arterial obstruction by the cannula is compounded by the diversion of blood through the circuit.

Using a pumpless arterio-venous system introduces a new vascular bed to the patient. The heart has to pump blood through the brain, liver, kidneys and other organs and the membrane of the ECCO$_2$R.

Veno-venous ECCO$_2$R

Veno-venous ECCO$_2$R systems utilize a pump to generate flow across a membrane.

Single-site venous cannulation is possible, as low flow allows the use of smaller cannulas, even if they contain both the drainage and return lumens.

The set-up is then very similar to RRT, and indeed some systems are trying to combine the two into one. These developments are, however, impeded by a higher risk of thrombosis and circuit obstruction.

These systems allow easy mobilization of the patient.

Complications of ECCO$_2$R

Similar issues to those observed on ECMO are possible.

Distal limb ischaemia due to arterial cannulation is the main risk in veno-arterial ECCO$_2$R. Compartment syndrome of the lower limb requiring fasciotomy or limb amputation are devastating consequences.

Haemorrhage is the most commonly reported complication in ECCO$_2$R. The low blood flow renders systemic anticoagulation mandatory, and this increases the risk of significant bleeding including cerebral, gastrointestinal and nasopharyngeal bleeds. Conversely, thrombus formation with clots detaching and entering the patient's bloodstream, plugging the membrane or obstructing the cannula lumen will be seen when anticoagulation is not achieved.

Heparin-induced thrombocytopenia and thrombocytopenia (see Chapter 7) are commonly observed.

Bleeding and infection at the cannulation sites are possible.

Clinical management

Anticoagulation

The same principles apply for ECCO$_2$R as for ECMO (see Chapter 7), except that a higher degree of anticoagulation is often required as the blood flow in the ECCO$_2$R circuit is usually lower than in the ECMO circuit.

Circuit monitoring

The primary goal in monitoring the circuit is to prevent emergencies and patient complications.

Blood flows, gas sweep and the amount of CO$_2$ removal (when available) should be documented hourly.

Blood flow across the circuit can be monitored continuously using an ultrasonic flow probe. Low flows are associated with increased risk of clotting in the circuit and oxygenator and with inefficient removal of CO$_2$. Low flows may be caused by kinked tubing or thrombi developing in the system.

Removal of CO$_2$ can be measured by sampling the blood before and after the membrane. Some systems measure CO$_2$ removal automatically. As for ECMO, water vapour will build up on the membrane and reduce gas transfer. This requires a regular blast of air across the membrane to drain the water out.

Any visible clot should be noted. The circuit and pump should be checked regularly for development of thrombi and the position documented; this is of particular importance if the clot or fibrin strands are noted close to the return cannula.

Distal limb observations should be documented hourly to allow early detection of poor blood flow and prevent complications of ischaemia.

Cannula sites should be checked regularly, noting any signs of infection or bleeding. Adequate fixation of the cannula should be checked regularly to prevent accidental decannulation. The circuit tubing should be secured and the skin protected from potential pressure of heavy tubing.

Patient management

All principles are identical to those used in ECMO patients.

Liberation from ECCO$_2$R

Liberation from ECCO$_2$R should be considered as soon as the patient can maintain appropriate PaCO$_2$ levels without relying on harmful positive-pressure ventilation.

A trial off sweep gas should be attempted daily.

Key points

- CO$_2$ clearance is achieved with lower blood flow through the circuit.
- ECCO$_2$R allows a decrease in the insult of mechanical ventilation (least-damaging lung ventilation).

TO LEARN MORE

Health Quality Ontario. (2010). Extracorporeal lung support technologies – bridge to recovery and bridge to lung transplantation in adult patients: an evidence-based analysis. *Ontario Health Technology Assessment Series*, 10, 1–47.

Moerer O, Quintel M. (2011). Protective and ultra-protective ventilation: using pumpless interventional lung assist (iLA). *Minerva Anestesiologica*, 77, 537–44.

Terragni P, Maiolo G, Ranieri VM. (2012). Role and potentials of low-flow CO$_2$ removal system in mechanical ventilation. *Current Opinion in Critical Care*, 18, 93–8.

Chapter 14

ECMO to support organ donation

Many patients listed for transplantation will die before receiving an organ or become too ill for transplantation. The donor pool could be expanded by aggressive physiological support of marginal brain-dead donors or organ donation after cardiac death (DCD).

Organ ischaemia is the most important factor decreasing organ quality in DCD and some marginal brain-dead donors. Optimization of therapeutic support to maintain solid organ perfusion and oxygenation can be achieved with ECMO.

ECMO as a bridge for organ donation in brain-dead donors

Retrieval of organs often fails in brain-dead donors due to the inability to provide physiological support before, during and after the declaration of death.

Invasive haemodynamic monitoring, administration of vasoactive drugs and steroids, and hormone-replacement therapy in the potential donor are often insufficient to achieve the goals required for a safe organ procurement.

Instituting veno-arterial ECMO in unstable brain-dead donors allows organ support.

If instituted before the diagnosis of brain death, standard tests cannot be conducted. For example, the apnoea test has to be modified and requires decreasing the sweep gas flow to allow a significant rise in $PaCO_2$.

ECMO as a bridge for organ donation in non-heart-beating donors

Non-heart-beating or DCD donors are those who die after unsuccessful cardiac resuscitation.

Uncontrolled donors have suffered an incident in the community with subsequent admission to hospital. Controlled donors are patients with brain injury deemed irreversible who have not met the criteria for brain death. Donation will follow withdrawal of treatment.

In addition to ethical considerations, deceased cardiac donors are currently under-used because of concerns about poor rates of graft survival due to longer periods of warm ischaemia. Livers obtained in these conditions have a worse outcome, although it does not appear to have a great effect on the kidneys, lungs and pancreas.

Early reperfusion with ECMO could improve the viability of the organs, increasing the potential donor pool.

Post-mortem in vivo organ preservation with chest compressions, mechanical ventilation and ECMO for uncontrolled DCD programmes has been successfully implemented in some countries. This involves transfer of the potential DCD donor to the hospital and starting femora–femoral veno-arterial partial extracorporeal support with deep hypothermia for the preservation of abdominal cavity organs while waiting family consent.

Controlled donors allow rapid institution of veno-arterial ECMO after death has been declared, and this is now used to retrieve hearts that have subsequently been implanted successfully. Ethical implications need to be addressed at a national level and local guidance adhered to.

TO LEARN MORE

Shemie SD. (2014). Life, death, and the bridges in-between. *Annals of the New York Academy of Sciences*, 1330, 101–4.

Chapter 15

ECMO registries and research

ECMO is an extraordinary technique applied to a small number of patients. Registries are useful in these circumstances to ensure that experience and learning can be shared among many clinicians.

The Extracorporeal Life Support Organization registry

The ELSO maintains a data registry. This was started in 1989 (see Chapter 1: In the beginning), but data goes back to 1976. It has more than 100 centres contributing data. It was initially essentially paediatric.

Data entry is voluntary but requires adhesion as a member. Members pay an annual fee that allows them to enter data and receive regular reports, including comparison of outcomes with similar centres.

The registry summarises cumulative experience, is open for individual queries about specific patient outcomes, supports observational studies and allows benchmarking.

International ECMO Network

The International ECMO Network (ECMONet) is dedicated to conducting and supporting high-quality, high-impact research aimed at defining the role of extracorporeal life support in the management of respiratory and cardiac failure in adults, helping to build on the scientific foundation for its use and driving continuous improvement in its application where appropriate.

ECMONet is committed to a collaborative vision of scientific research in the field, one in which investigators from around the world may propose and lead projects, with the Network simply soliciting and prioritizing studies, and facilitating clinical trials.

TO LEARN MORE

Extracorporeal Life Support Organization
(https://www.elso.org).
International ECMO Network
(http://www.internationalecmonetwork.org/).

APPENDIX: THE FUTURE OF ECMO

It is impossible to predict the future!

In 1980, no one could have predicted how ubiquitous the mobile phone would be or how ECMO would be used to support an ever-increasing number of patients.

The immediate future of ECMO, or the now, is about limiting its complications by improving the design of circuits and cannula, and sharing practice and experience between clinicians.

Key elements of ECMO support are an understanding of which patients should be supported and their management while they are supported, and to acknowledge that some patients will not benefit from support on ECMO.

ECMO support is often the last option, and progress should aim at understanding how to prevent and treat those conditions leading to this support being required.

The ECMO technician will continue to strive to improve ECMO, while the ECMO clinicians' aim will be to find what is needed to avoid ECMO!

INDEX